Development of
Indices of

ACCESS TO
MEDICAL CARE

Development of Indices of

ACCESS TO
MEDICAL CARE

Lu Ann Aday
Ronald Andersen

Health Administration Press
Ann Arbor

*Published with the support of
the Robert Wood Johnson Foundation*

Health Administration Press
M2240 School of Public Health
The University of Michigan
Ann Arbor, Michigan 48104
(313) 764-1380

Contents

Foreword

In developing its initial national program, The Robert Wood Johnson Foundation elected to place major emphasis on improving access to ambulatory health care for the citizens of the United States. Thus, in our grant making efforts to date, we have given intensive study to programs designed to strengthen, or improve, or recast the kinds of front-line medical care traditionally provided by out-of-hospital physicians.

As we have gotten more deeply involved in this program, it has become increasingly evident that although there are many heartrending testimonials about the difficulties which individual Americans experience in getting help from a doctor, there is a distressing lack of solid information about the magnitude of the problem, its distribution, or the actual numbers of people who are experiencing trouble in obtaining satisfactory personal medical help when they need it.

Historically, policy makers have used a crude proxy measure of this problem. This has been the ratio of the number of physicians to the number of people in a particular geographic area. Where the ratio has been found to be low, it has been assumed that people have trouble in securing physician services; where it is found to be high, it has been assumed that the ambulatory medical care needs of people were probably being handled satisfactorily. While these ratios have been useful gross guidelines for overall planning, they are simply not sensitive or sophisticated enough to really give the information needed for long range planning for a better delivery system. Further, the presence of high-speed transportation systems, or super highways, or extensive telephone communication lines, or regional hospital outpatient departments, or varying mixes of general physicians to physician specialists in different areas make just the number of physicians in a particular locale a most inadequate index on which to make judgments about the difficulty a particular patient or a particular community is having in obtaining adequate physician care.

Despite this absence of any reliable measuring rod, large amounts of governmental and philanthropic funds have been devoted to developing new kinds of health professionals, increasing America's output of physicians, and experimenting with new ways of delivering basic health services. While these are laudatory efforts, their impact is hard to evaluate when baseline information against which national or local progress can be measured is lacking.

It is thus our belief, a belief shared by many, that we must have some better indicators which, through periodic surveys, can measure more precisely just how hard it is to get needed physician care if our national efforts to improve the availability of medical services are to be properly assessed. Development of such indicators could provide a baseline to determine the nation's progress toward providing more satisfactory entry into the personal medical care system, and will be important to all funding agencies, to our foundation, and to others working in this area of critical social concern.

Thus, The Robert Wood Johnson Foundation is pleased to have been able to provide assistance for the preparation and publication of this particular study. The work, entitled *Access to Medical Care,* represents a thoughtful attempt to examine both conceptually and practically what kinds of information could tell us more accurately and precisely the problems people face in obtaining physician care in different parts of the country.

From the Foundation's perspective, we hope to be able to use the proposed access-to-care index as one of the basic tools in the Foundation's evaluation of its own activities in this area. We also feel that this study, and those which will follow from the Center for Health Administration Studies at the University of Chicago, will be useful to other health professionals, scholars, and planners interested in one of America's current social problems — that of delivering effective, dignified, and humane care to all of the people in our large and diverse country.

David E. Rogers, M.D.
Princeton, New Jersey
October, 1974

Preface

One of the major difficulties in formulating a rational health service delivery system is the paucity of performance indicators which are sufficiently specific so that a particular model can be constructed with known inputs and outputs. Given the state of the art of measurable performance indicators, public policy formulation takes the form of balancing off public demand, supply, and amount of money — as exemplified by a variety of existing health service delivery systems. Each system claims it is performing at a certain net level of results without being able to demonstrate that it is so doing — with the exception of the amount of money it is costing.

During the last thirty years or so, however, there is one performance indicator — and measurable — which is getting increasing attention because of the public policy of equalizing access to health services, regardless of income and residence, for example. This performance indicator is the nature of public access to the health services system. Any access indicator should serve the purpose of measuring the extent to which income groups vary in their ease of entry to the system, for example. That indicator should also attempt to measure how the need for care and the services received for it are related.

This project is an attempt to explore and formulate indicators of access to health services which can be applied to health services delivery systems with a variety of objectives and in a range of circumstances. The development of such performance indicators should assist in measuring the convenience, appropriateness to medical need and (emotional, financial, etc.) costs of gaining "access" to the health care system.

Odin W. Anderson
October, 1974

Acknowledgements

Numerous people have been involved and contributed to the efforts reported here.

We wish to acknowledge our appreciation to the Robert Wood Johnson Foundation, which provided the grant through which this study was financed. Robert Blendon of the Johnson Foundation was especially helpful in suggesting how we might incorporate the immediate concerns of the Foundation into our general approach to the access concept.

We appreciate the efforts of Joel May in drafting the original proposal to the Foundation. Special thanks go to other members of the Center for Health Administration Studies staff who provided useful feedback on our approach, especially Steve Shortell whose conceptual and administrative support throughout the course of the study has greatly enriched the efforts reported here.

We wish to express our appreciation, also, to our numerous consultants from the following agencies or institutions: the American Hospital Association, American Medical Association, Health Services Research and Training Program (Purdue University), Center for Medical Sociology and Health Services Research (University of Wisconsin), Department of Medical Care and Hospitals (Johns Hopkins University), Measuring Health Concepts Research Testing Center (Southern Illinois University), Bureau of Health Services Research and Evaluation, National Center for Health Statistics and the Social Security Administration. The feedback and suggestions from health services research professionals at each of these institutions was of invaluable assistance in helping us refine our approach to the access concept.

We wish to also thank Gretchen Voorhis Fleming, Madeline Mirabito and David Garth Taylor, who helped carry out the analyses reported here and did much of the "leg work" to glean information on the access concept from the literature and extant data sources.

Thanks go also to Evelyn Friedman and Linda Randall, who typed the original manuscript for this volume and to Grace Chiu and Elaine Scheye, who helped edit it.

Lu Ann Aday
Ronald Andersen

Authors'
Introductory Notes

In early 1973 the research staff of the Center for Health Administration Studies (CHAS) submitted a research application to the Robert Wood Johnson Foundation entitled, "Development of an Index of Access to Health Care." The project was funded and work began in April, 1973. By the end of October, 1973, a preliminary report was completed which documented our conceptual scheme, empirical efforts, and plans for the remainder of the year.*

This volume is based on the final report to the Foundation of our first year's work on this project. It elaborates the ideas and further develops the analyses suggested in the preliminary report and points out the directions the project will move in the second year.

The discussion that follows is divided into two main sections: (1) a conceptual and empirical overview of access, and (2) a research appendix containing abstracts of selected references relevant to access and descriptions of existing data sources in which information on aspects of access have been collected.

The first section is divided into four main parts. Chapter 1 presents our theoretical framework for the study of the access concept. Chapter 2 presents analyses of selected process and outcome indices of access, based on data collected in the 1970 Center for Health Administration Studies nationwide survey of health services utilization and expenditures. Chapter 3 documents the methods used in the study. Chapter 4 is a

*The Preliminary Report was entitled "Development of a Framework for the Study of Access to Health Care," by L.A. Aday, et al., Center for Health Administration Studies, University of Chicago (October, 1973).

comprehensive overview of the literature relevant to the access concept.

The Research Appendix has two main parts. The first part contains 125 abstracts of selected references relevant to the access concept. These abstracts emphasize recent works which have been published subsequent to a literature review of utilization studies published by the Bureau of Health Services Research and Evaluation (Aday and Eichhorn, 1972). The second part contains description and evaluation of data sources judged to be most relevant to construct and update national measure of access.

In the coming year, we plan to draw upon the work documented in this volume to complete our evaluations of various access measures and to refine our conceptual approach. We also plan to do a pilot study and pretest a questionnaire designed to collect information from a national sample of the population needed to operationalize the measures of access we have developed. Finally, a design will be developed which (1) outlines a national study of access to medical care, tentatively scheduled to be carried out in a third year of the project, and (2) incorporates plans to assess levels of access and change in access over time at the community level. The purpose of the latter endeavor is to provide one mechanism for evaluating the impact of delivery programs funded by the Johnson Foundation in various communities around the country.

Tables

Figures

1

A Framework for the Study of Access To Medical Care

Statement of the Problem

Health care policy makers, planners and administrators and the medical care consumer himself are increasingly voicing their concern that access to the medical care system should be improved. A plethora of programs have subsequently been launched during the past decade with the expressed objective of improving equity of access to medical care in the United States.

Some of these programs are directed at increasing the buying power or medical know-how of the health care consumer — Medicaid, Medicare, national health insurance and health education or nutrition programs, respectively. Others seek to improve the availability or organization of medical manpower and facilities — development of family practice specialty, paramedical training programs, Health Maintenance Organizations, etc.

All of these programs are intended in some way to enhance equity of access to the medical care system for various groups in the population. Just what the concept of access means, however, much less how it might be measured and what methods should be used to evaluate it are ill-defined at present. Thus far, access has been more of a political than an operational idea. It has for some time been an expressed or at least implicit goal of health policy. However, few attempts have been made to provide formalized conceptual or empirical definitions of access that permit policy makers and consumers to actually monitor the effectiveness of various programs in meeting that goal.

The purpose of this report is to correct some of these deficiencies in the conceptualization and measurement of access. Two primary objectives subsequently characterize this introductory theoretical section: 1) to present a framework for the study of the access concept, and 2) to suggest how alternative empirical definitions of access might be constructed.

Background Literature

DEFINITIONS AND INDICES OF ACCESS

Two main themes regarding the access concept appear in the literature. Some researchers tend to equate access with characteristics of the population (family income, insurance coverage, attitudes toward medical care) or of the delivery system — the distribution and organization of manpower and facilities, for example. Others argue that access can best be evaluated through outcome indicators of the individual's passage through the system, such as utilization rates or satisfaction scores. Representatives of both schools of thought will be summarized here.

A U.S. Department of Agriculture (U.S.D.A.) report on the problems of health services in rural areas concludes, for example, that:

> . . . rural and urban people do not have equal access to health services. Rural areas are deficient in professional medical personnel, physical health care facilities, and the ability to afford the financial costs of illness (U.S.D.A., 1973:23).

In the U.S.D.A. report then, access means the availability of financial and health system resources in an area.

Bodenheimer (1970) and Freeborn and Greenlick (1973) emphasize that "access" assumes services are available whenever and wherever the patient needs them and that the system point of entry is well-defined.

Chen (1973), in a first attempt to develop explicit quantifiable indicators of access, introduces two descriptive indices of the actual organization and availability of services. One index is a weighted sum of the appointment waiting time, travel time, waiting room time and actual processing time for the patients in a given medical care facility and a second is intended to reflect the difference between the ideal and actual number of services, personnel or equipment in a given community.

Rogers (1973) points out that a decline in the number and availability of primary care physicians inhibits the access of medical care consumers to the system. Gibson, et al. (1970), for example, report that hospital emergency rooms are increasingly becoming centers for the receipt of primary care. They cite the decline of primary practitioners due to specialization, the reluctance of physicians to make house calls and unavailability of private physicians in the urban inner-city to account for this trend.

Donabedian (1973) describes two main aspects of accessibility — socio-organizational and geographic. Socio-organizational attributes include all those attributes of the resources that either facilitate or hinder the efforts of the client to reach care — other than spatial attributes. This would include such things as the sex of the provider, his fee scale and specialization, etc. Geographic accessibility, on the other hand, refers to the friction of space that is a function of the time and physical distance that must be traversed to get care.

Mechanic (1972), however, in considering the factors that influence the utilization of health services points out that the availability of services and resources is not enough to account for entry or non-entry to the system. One must also consider the potential consumer's willingness to seek care. This characteristic depends on his health attitudes, knowledge about health care and the social and cultural definitions of illness he has learned.

Further, Shortell (1973) takes issue with characterizations of access itself as descriptive properties of individuals or the delivery system. The problem in looking at access in terms of criteria such as cost, availability, internal economy (waiting time, delays and interruptions in receiving services, etc.), psychological variables or health knowledge, he argues, is that in themselves, they do not tell us whether people who want to get in the system actually do or not. He asserts that there should be some type of external validation of whether these factors make a difference with respect to getting care, such as examining the utilization rates over time for groups that possess these properties.

Somers, in a discussion of the health care crisis in the United States, points out:

A considerable part of the problem . . . is the fact that so many people still lack access to good health care. For many, it is quantitatively deficient. For many more, including many in middle and upper-income categories, it is qualitatively lacking, particularly in the educational influence of a good doctor-patient relationship, a lack that probably disturbs the patient even more than it does the doctor (Somers, 1971:23).

Implicit in the characterizations of access as properties of the individual or the system then is the assumption, as Somers suggests, that the quantity and quality of an individual's passage through the medical care system is affected by these factors.

A number of indices appear in the literature that reflect quantitative or qualitative outcome dimensions of access.

Fox (1972), for example, argues that financing and supply factors are the main barriers to access and that the actual access rates are best gauged by the utilization for designated populations or subgroups.

Some researchers emphasize the access concept is best considered in the context of whether the people actually in need of medical care receive it or not. Beck (1973), for example, uses a "medical iceberg" notion to conceptualize access. The iceberg itself represents the set of medical needs that might be treated by a physician. The proportion of the iceberg above water represents those needs which actually receive the attention of a physician. The greater the portion of the iceberg above water, the greater the access to care of the group represented by that iceberg. Freeborn and Greenlick (1973) also suggest that "accessibility" implies that people in the population-at-risk use services at rates proportional and appropriate to their existing need for care. The Bureau of Health Services Research and Evaluation (BHSRE) has developed a need-based empirical indicator of the access concept — the use-disability ratio (the number of physician visits per 100 days of disability experienced) — that explicitly operationalizes this consideration of access as the use of services by the population-at-risk relative to their expressed need for care (Health Services Research and Training Program, 1972).

Shortell (1973) introduces several "continuity-access indices" — the number of different providers seen to get an illness episode resolved, the number of visits to each provider, and the reason or source of referral to each provider — that reflect both the volume and pattern of the process of care-seeking.

Andersen, et al. (1971) report subjective consumer evaluations of accessibility gauged by their satisfaction with their waiting time in doctors' offices, the availability of care at night and on weekends, and the ease and convenience of getting a doctor. Freeborn and Greenlick (1973) assert that satisfaction with the accessibility of care can be evaluated by the patient's attitudes regarding the extent to which services are available at the time and place needed and whether the person perceived a change in his condition as a result of care.

In summary, a variety of definitions and indicators of access appear in the literature. Some research implies that access is a function of the characteristics of the delivery system or the population. Indices of access, for this group, are simply descriptors of the organization or availability of care or the attitudes or resources of potential consumers. A second body of research suggests that access is best evaluated by outcome indicators of the rate or quality of passage through the system, such as utilization rates or satisfaction scores. These measures, they argue, permit external validation of the importance of the system and individual characteristics.

A SOCIAL INDICATOR FRAMEWORK FOR THE STUDY OF ACCESS

Over the past decade, Congress, HEW, social scientists and others have directed their attention to the construction of social indicators of the quality of life in the United States, that would be analogous to the economic indicators of the nation's financial well-being (Wilcox et al., 1972). Access to medical care, too, might be considered a kind of social indicator of the process and behavioral and subjective outcomes of individuals' entry to the medical care system. In the discussion that follows, the contribution of social indicators research to providing a framework for the study of the access concept will be examined.

Kenneth Land (1972) points out that to understand how desired outcomes in a social system might be achieved, it is necessary to specify what the expressed objectives or end-points are and, also, a conceptual model of how the various determinants of these outcomes relate to one another and the desired end-points. The outcomes, he says, are output-type social indicators and the predictor variables analytic social indicators. Roos (1973), in presenting a model to evaluate program effectiveness, calls these indicators impact and process evaluative criteria, respectively.

James Coleman (1971) carries this theme forward when he argues that in policy research, one must actually consider three types of variables. There are outcome variables, that are output-type indicators or dependent variables. In addition, there are two types of independent or analytic variables, *policy* variables, which can be or have been amenable to policy and *control* variables that affect the outcome variables, but themselves, cannot be changed by public policy.

The focus upon the more processual (or independent) variables versus the outcome-type measures in any effort to evaluate access itself depends on — in the language of evaluation research — whether one is primarily concerned with the goals (or outcomes) of the delivery system itself or with how the system and the participants in the system interact to achieve these objectives, i.e., with a goal attainment or systems-type evaluation model.

The research on the utilation of health services suggests important dependent and manipulable (policy) and non-manipulable (control) independent variables that might be incorporated into a framework for the study of access to health care. The formal definition of access itself implies an approach to or use of a given service or object and the factors that affect or impede this process. Webster, for example, defines access as "permission, liberty, or ability to enter, approach, communicate with, or pass to and from or to make use of." Health services utilization research, provides a framework to describe those factors that inhibit or facilitate entrance to the health delivery system, measurements of where, how often and for what purposes entry is gained, and how these inhibiting (or facilitating) factors operate to affect admittance. In the section that follows, the literature on the predictors and indices of health services utilization will be placed within the social indicators and policy research perspectives just summarized, to articulate our theoretical perspective for the study of access.

A Framework for the Study of Access

The basic framework for the access concept presented here is drawn from the social indicators and policy research perspectives just reviewed, the utilization literature and the existing material on access itself as a concept (see Figure 1).

DEFINITIONS OF CONCEPTS

Health Policy

Access has been most often considered in a political context. Improved access to care is an important goal of much of health policy. Numerous financing, education, manpower and health care reorganization programs, for example, have been introduced with this objective in mind. It may be well then to characterize health policy as the starting point for consideration of the access concept. It is the effect of health policy on altering access to medical care that health planners and policy makers are often concerned with evaluating.

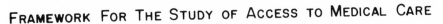

FIGURE I
FRAMEWORK FOR THE STUDY OF ACCESS TO MEDICAL CARE

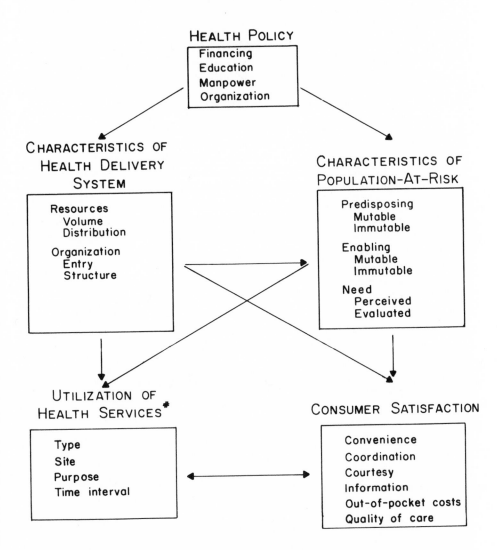

#Type — hospital, physician, dentist, drug other
 Site — physician's office, clinic, hospital inpatient, outpatient, emergency room, other
 Purpose — preventive, illness-related (curative or stabilizing), custodial
 Time interval — contact, volume, continuity

Characteristics of Health Delivery System

The components of the health delivery system in Figure 1 are, in general, those specified by Andersen, et al. (1970) for the health services system. The term "delivery system" is used to refer more specifically to those arrangements for the potential rendering of care to consumers.

The delivery system is characterized by two main elements — resources and organization. Resources are the labor and capital devoted to health care. Included would be health personnel, structures in which health care and education are provided, and the equipment and materials used in providing health services. The resources component includes both the volume and distribution of medical resources in an area.

Organization describes "what the system does with its resources. It refers to the manner in which medical personnel and facilities are coordinated and controlled in the process of providing medical services." The components of organization are entry and structure. Entry refers to the process of gaining entrance to the system (travel time, waiting time, etc.). (Andersen et al., 1970, term this component "access" and define it as the "means through which the patient gains entry to the medical care system and continues the treatment process.") Structure, the second component of organization, concerns "the characteristics of the system that determine what happens to the patient following entry to the system" (whom he sees, how he is treated).

The characteristics of the delivery system are aggregate, structural properties. The system or a particular delivery organization is the unit of analysis, rather than the individual.

The resources and organization of the system, as defined here, embody the characterizations of access as a system property that appear in the literature.

Characteristics of Population-at-Risk

The characteristics of the population-at-risk are the predisposing, enabling and need components that Andersen and Newman (1973) describe as the individual determinants of utilization.

The predisposing component includes those variables that describe the propensity of individuals to use services. These properties exist prior to the onset of illness episodes. They include such things as age, sex, race, religion and values concerning health and illness.

The enabling component describes the means individuals have available to them for the use of services. Both resources specific to the individual and his family (income, insurance coverage) and attributes of the community in which the individual lives (rural-urban character, region) are included here.

Need refers to illness level, which is the most immediate cause of health service use. The need for care may be either perceived by the individual or evaluated by the delivery system.

In considering the population-at-risk, an individual rather than the system is the elemental unit of analysis. Similar information may be collected to describe the population-at-risk and the delivery system (rural-urban residence, solo or group practice plan, waiting time, etc.). Computation and interpretation of the indices themselves, however, depend on whether individuals or the delivery system is the elemental object of study. The household survey is the best method for collecting data on the population-at-risk. When a community or a specific delivery organization is the object of concern, the Census, manpower data, or clinic records may be the best sources of information.

Implicit in the access concept is the fact that certain categories of people have more or less "access" to medical care than others. The characteristics, which are biological or social "givens," such as one's age, sex, or race (that appear as predisposing variables) or some of the community characteristics (urban-rural) in the enabling component, serve to define these groups. The more manipulable beliefs and enabling variables, such as income or health insurance coverage, are characteristics which health policy seeks to change, in order to affect these groups' access to care. The more manipulable components, Andersen and Newman term "mutable" variables, the less manipulable "immutable."

Utilization of Health Services

Implied in the review of the literature on the access concept is that there should be some external validation of the effect of these characteristics of the population-at-risk and of the delivery system on people's entry (or non-entry) to the system. The level and pattern of the population's actual utilization of the system is one measure that may be used to test the predictive validity of these system- and individual-based access indicators.

The utilization of health services may be characterized in terms of the type, site, purpose or time interval of use.

The type of utilization means whether it was a unit of hospital, physician, dentist, etc. use (Anderson, 1963). This category refers to the kind of service received and who provided it.

Consumers complain that it is becoming more and more difficult to find a primary care physician who will give them the personal attention they want. It seems relevant, then, in operationalizing the access concept, to specify what types of providers actually do render services to consumers.

The site of the medical care encounter refers to the place where care was received: doctor's office, hospital outpatient department, emergency room, etc.

Patients also express the concern that physicians no longer make house calls and that they have to go to hospital emergency rooms for treatment after the doctor's regular office hours. It is important in evaluating access, to know where the majority of people actually do go to have their medical needs met.

The purpose of a visit means whether it was for preventive, illness-related or custodial care. Preventive care refers to efforts to stop illness before it begins — e.g., checkups, immunizations. Illness-related care may be either curative or stabilizing. Curative care means "the process of treatment which returns an individual to his previous state of functioning." It most often refers to the treatment of acute illnesses. Stabilizing care provides "stabilization for long-term irreversible (chronic) illness such as heart disease or diabetes." Custodial care provides mainly for the personal needs of the patient, but makes no effort to treat his underlying illness conditions. It is the care provided mainly in nursing homes and extended care facilities. These three different reasons or purposes for care seeking — preventive, illness-related, or custodial — imply distinctly different patterns of care seeking. It is important, in conceptualizing access, to be able to specify the kinds of demands placed on the system by those who would seek to gain entrance to it.

The time interval for a visit may be expressed in terms of contact, volume, or continuity measures. Contact refers to whether or not the person entered the medical care system in a given period of time. In describing access, policy makers are concerned with who gets into the system, but more especially, those who do not. Volume refers to the number of contacts and revisits in a given time interval. This measure reflects who gets into the system and how often he uses it. Continuity refers to the degree of linkage and coordination of medical services associated with a particular illness experience or episode. Consumers complain that the process of receiving care is fragmented and poorly organized, and therefore, people lack appropriate access to the system. The continuity dimension of the utilization concept permits these level-of-integration aspects of the process of obtaining medical care to be operationalized.

It is important to specify the relevant dimension of utilization. Each reflects different aspects of the care-seeking process. Further the impact of the various determinants of utilization may vary, depending on the type, site, purpose or time interval analyzed.

Consumer Satisfaction

Consumer satisfaction refers to the attitudes of those who have experienced a contact with the medical care system toward the system. It is different from the medical beliefs component of the predisposing variables in that it measures users' satisfaction with the quantity or quality of care actually received. Medical beliefs refer to diffuse sociocultural predispositions toward health and medicine. Consumer satisfaction, however, is probably best evaluated in the context of a specific, recent and identifiable episode of medical care seeking. Dimensions of satisfaction that seem relevant to consider in eliciting subjective perceptions of access are satisfaction with the convenience of care, its coordination, the courtesy shown by providers, information given to the patient concerning how he should deal with his illness, the out-of-pocket costs required for care and the quality of care he thinks he received.

THE FRAMEWORK

The preceding discussion has provided a description of the elements it is relevant to consider in operationalizing the access concept. The framework in Figure 1 also points out the hypothesized relationships among these different components. The implication of the arrows in Figure 1 is, for example, that health policy may be intended to directly affect characteristics of the delivery system, such as increasing the supply of physicians in an area. Or, programs may be directed to changing characteristics of the population-at-risk either directly (insurance coverage, education) or through the delivery system (facilities may be relocated, thereby reducing the travel time to care of area residents). Some properties of the population-at-risk are capable of being altered by health policy (mutable), while others are not (immutable). The latter characteristics are more properly considered delineators of groups for whom access differs than descriptors of access *per se*.

The delivery system may attempt to directly affect utilization patterns and satisfaction of the consumers with system. These effects are determined by the structure itself and not necessarily mediated by the properties of potential users. For example, members of group practice plans are found to have lower hospitalization rates than solo, fee-for-service plan users. This difference seems to persist, independent of the characteristics of consumers. One would be especially interested in these direct effects of system properties, when doing system-level analyses, with the system or organization itself as the elemental unit of concern rather than the population-at-risk — as for example, when comparing the effects of different health care delivery models on enrollee satisfaction and use.

On the other hand, the characteristics of the population itself (attitudes toward medical care, income, etc.) may directly affect use and satisfaction, independent of system properties. These are the relationships reported most often in social survey research on the utilization of services by a population of potential consumers.

Further, the system may also impact on the characteristics of the population and thereby indirectly affect its utilization of services and the consumer's satisfaction with care, as through effective public health education programs.

The double-headed arrow between utilization and satisfaction in Figure 1 suggests a sequence, over time, where the utilization of services is apt to influence a consumer's satisfaction with the system and, in turn, the satisfaction or dissatisfaction he experiences from this encounter influences his subsequent use of services.

Indices of Access

Two main categories of social indicators of the access concept may be specified, based on the framework just presented — process and outcome indices.

The process indices refer to the independent variables or predictors of the outcome of health policy. They reflect characteristics of the delivery system and the population-at-risk that affect whether entry to the system is gained and how satisfied consumers are with it. These process measures may be further classified according to their degree of manipulability by health policy. Mutable properties are ones that health policy seeks to alter, in the short run, to affect the utilization of or satisfaction with care (medical manpower distribution, insurance coverage, etc.). They are more meaningfully considered social indicators of the access concept, than the immutable properties, which serve more to define subgroups or target populations to whom health policy should be directed, i.e., age, sex, race, residence groups, for whom access differs.

The outcome indices are the dependent variables, the end-products of health policy regarding access. These measures include both objective and subjective descriptors of the population's entry to and passage through the system, i.e., utilization and satisfaction indices, respectively.

Summary

The purpose of the preceding discussion has been two-fold: (1) to present a framework for the study of access-to-medical care; and (2) to suggest how alternative empirical definitions of access might be derived from it.

Health policy was introduced as the starting point, for consideration of the access concept, for it is the impact of health policy on access to care that policy makers and administrators are most concerned with evaluating. Health policy is intended to affect both the characteristics of the delivery system (the volume and distribution of its resources and how it is organized) and the population-at-risk (through public education or financing programs, for example). These changes, in turn, ultimately influence people's utilization of services and how satisfied they are with the care they receive.

To most effectively evaluate the progress of health policy toward achieving the equity of access objective, however, explicit empirical indicators of the access concept should be developed. Such indicators might focus on operationalizing the changes that take place in the delivery system (re-distribution of resources, for example) or the population itself (more positive attitudes toward preventive health practices or universal insurance coverage) as a function of health policy. Or, the measures may be designed to describe the effects of policy in people's utilization of services and the satisfaction with the care they receive. Those measures that describe more of the process of implementing policy objectives (in terms of system or individual changes) are termed "process" indices and the ones which summarize the effects of these changes on utilization and satisfaction are called "outcome" measures. Those process measures which are manipulable by public policy (mutable) are more explicit "social indicators" of the access concept than are the less manipulable (immutable) indices — age, sex, residence, etc. The latter serve more to define target groups for which "access" (scores on the outcome and *mutable* process measures) may differ.

The following quotation from Avedis Donabedian provides an apt summary of many of these concerns with respect to the conceptualization and measurement of access:

The proof of access is use of service, not simply the presence of a facility. Access can, accordingly, be measured by the level of use in relation to "need." One should recognize, however, that clients and professionals evaluate "need" differently. Further, one must distinguish two components in use of service: "initiation" and "continuation." This is because different factors influence each, though any one factor may influence both. It is hardly necessary to emphasize that barriers to access are not only financial but also psychological, informational, social, organizational, spatial, temporal and so on. (Donabedian, 1972:111)

It is perhaps most meaningful then to consider access in terms of whether those who need care get into the system or not. One must recognize, however, that patients' perceptions and practitioners' evaluations of need may differ. Further, though diverse factors may influence whether an individual enters the medical care system initially, the organization of the system to provide care and the consumer's level of satisfaction with it are apt to determine whether he continues to seek services. The factors that affect the behavioral (utilization) and subjective (satisfaction) outcomes of care-seeking may be properties of the individuals themselves or of the medical care system they seek to enter. A framework concerned with evaluating access should identify what these factors are and the potential conceptual and empirical importance of each.

2
Process and Outcome Indicators of Access

Introduction

This section presents empirical analyses of some important process and outcome indices of access. All of the analyses were based on the 1970 Center for Health Administration Studies (CHAS) survey (See Chapter 3 for a description of the sample design).

A description of each index and the findings from the 1970 survey on it are presented. At the end of the discussion of the process and outcome measures, a summary of the findings and an evaluation of each index — in terms of its validity, reliability, variance, ease of collection, ease of computation, ease of interpretation and mutability — are provided.

Process Indices of Access

Process indices, as suggested in the theoretical discussion of the access concept, refer to characteristics of the delivery system or characteristics of the population-at-risk that affect people's utilization of and satisfaction with care. Information on these process indices may be collected and reported for the delivery system or a specific delivery organization, or they may be derived from data gathered from a survey of individuals, in the population-at-risk. An example of reporting a process index for a specific delivery organization would be the mean number of minutes a patient must wait before he sees a doctor in the facility, based on clinic logs, etc. The same information could be elicited from surveys of individuals in the population-at-risk, i.e., "How many minutes do you generally wait in your doctor's office before seeing him?" Collecting data on the delivery organization itself permits different systems to be compared, according to their "accessibility" on this particular aspect of the process of "entry" to the system. Reporting the mean office waiting time for persons in the population-at-risk permits those individuals and subgroups who have long waits to be identified, and the impact of this particular barrier on their satisfaction with and subsequent decisions to seek care, to be explored.

Some of the process indices that are relevant to consider in evaluating access are judged more susceptible to alteration by health policy (mutable) than others (immutable). The immutable properties of the population-at-risk (age, sex, race and residence, for example) identify groups or target populations who may differ in terms of their waiting times, and use patterns. The mutable descriptors of the delivery system or population — income, insurance coverage, whether or not one has a regular source of care, waiting time, for example — are properties that health policy seeks to alter to affect these groups' use of and satisfaction with care.

In the sections that follow, selected process indices of access will be introduced and the distribution of values on them for both manipulable (income and regular source of care) and non-manipulable (age, sex, race and residence) properties of a national sample of the population-at-risk will be introduced. The implication is that some groups have more access to care, based on these indices, than others. The purpose of the preliminary analyses of these indices is to begin to: (1) identify those groups for whom access differs; (2) evaluate the conceptual and methodological utility of these particular indices for detecting such differences; and (3) suggest how health policy might improve access.

The indices to be examined are as follows: regular source of care[1], travel time, appointment or walk-in visit, appointment waiting time and office waiting time.

---

[1]The regular source of care variable is used both as a dependent variable and as a mutable population descriptor (independent variable) in the analyses that follow.

REGULAR SOURCE OF CARE

Where people report they usually go when they are sick or want advice about their health influences whether or not they seek care. More importantly, once the decision to seek care is made, the regular source largely determines the type, site, volume and continuity of care the patient receives. Further, there is evidence that people who have a regular attending physician are more satisfied with the care they receive than those who do not have a particular place they can go when the need arises.

VARIABLE DESCRIPTION

The identification of the respondent's regular source of care was based on an inquiry about the "particular medical person or clinic (PERSON) usually goes to when sick or for advice about health." See Chapter 6, Data Source Evaluations, for a description of the 1970 CHAS survey on which these and subsequent analyses are based.

FINDINGS

Approximately 11 percent of the sample could identify no medical person or place that they went to for medical advice or treatment on a routine basis (See Table 1). The majority of the repondents reported they had a medical doctor — general practitioner or specialist — as their regular source of care. About 19 percent of the people indicated a clinic as their usual care source.

Children were least apt to report having no regular source of care. They were more likely to have clinics as their usual source of care, compared to the other age groups. Of those who reported a physician as their usual source, children were more apt to go to specialists than general practitioners. Children under the care of pediatricians probably account for this difference, since pediatricians are defined as specialists. Those age groups most likely to report no regular source of care were the young and middle-aged adults.

Males were somewhat less likely to report a regular source of care than females. Women were also more apt to have a specialist as a usual source than men. This difference is probably due to women having obstetrician-gynecologist-type practitioners (who are also defined as specialists) as their usual source of care.

Nonwhites, compared to whites, were less likely to have any regular source of care and more likely to use a clinic, if they reported a source at all.

The inner city and rural farm residents were most apt to have no

TABLE 1
Regular source of care(6) by selected characteristics of population-at-risk

	REGULAR SOURCE OF CARE(6)[a]				
CHARACTERISTIC	Percent none	Percent clinic	Percent GP	Percent specialist	TOTAL PERCENT
Age (1)					
1-5	6	22	38	34	100
6-17	8	21	47	24	100
18-34	14	19	45	23	101[b]
35-54	14	15	49	23	101[b]
55-64	13	17	47	23	100
65 and over	11	17	48	25	101[b]
Sex (2)					
Male	13	19	45	23	100
Female	9	18	46	26	99[b]
Race (3)					
White	10	17	47	26	100
Nonwhite	16	32	35	18	101[b]
Residence (4)					
SMSA, central city	15	24	35	26	100
SMSA, other urban	10	14	46	31	101[b]
Urban, non-SMSA	7	21	50	23	101[b]
Rural nonfarm	9	16	55	20	100
Rural farm	12	21	55	12	100
Poverty level (5)					
Above	9	16	47	28	100
Below	17	28	41	14	100
Total	11	19	46	25	100[b,c]

[a] In this and subsequent tables, numbers in parentheses after variable names refer to variable definitions given in Chapter 3. This table excludes people who reported some "other" source of care. These people constituted approximately four percent (4%) of the total U.S. population in 1970.

[b] Does not add up to 100 because of rounding error.

[c] Percent table N is of U.S. population equals 96; percent in "other" category or NA equals 4.

regular care source. Inner city dwellers were more apt to have clinics as their usual source of care than other city or rural residents. People who lived in rural areas were much more apt to have general practitioners as their regular attending physicians, while city dwellers outside the inner city were more apt to report specialists as their regular source of care.

People below the poverty level were almost twice as likely to report having no regular source of care than the nonpoor, or when they did have a regular care source, it was almost twice as apt to be a clinic. Further, people above the poverty level were much more likely to report having a specialist as their usual source of care than were the poor.

The meaning of "clinic" as a regular source of care varies considerably. Persons who use a hospital outpatient department or even an emergency room as their regular source of care will report that they use a clinic, as will members of a large prepaid group practice plan such as Kaiser or H.I.P., or users of a group of doctors in specialty practice. One way of differentiating care received by people who say they use a clinic is to ask if, within the institution where they obtain their regular care, they usually see the same doctor. Such information might be of particular value in assessing whether the patient feels comfortable about seeking care and the degree of continuity of care that he might receive.

Table 2 shows that there were considerable differences in the portions of people with a clinic as a regular source of care who saw a particular doctor. Older people and females were more likely to see a particular doctor, as were whites and the higher income groups. Urban dwellers in SMSA's were less likely to see a particular doctor than was the rest of the population.

The clinic care reported by the less advantaged portions of the population is apt to be the more depersonalized service provided in big city hospital emergency rooms and outpatient departments. The more well-off white segment is more likely to use a particular physician who may have some arrangement to combine his practice with other practitioners — through simply sharing the same facility or through more formalized partnerships or group practices. The fact that old people were much more apt to have a regular doctor when they use a clinic might be related to the financial impact of Medicare, which makes a private doctor possible for this group.

TRAVEL TIME TO CARE

There is evidence that the time that one must travel to obtain medical care affects the choice of the site where care is received. Further, some argue that the volume of services consumed is less for those who must travel long distances to care.

TABLE 2
Percent with clinic as regular source of care who usually see a particular doctor at clinic by selected characteristics of population-at-risk

	SEE PARTICULAR DOCTOR? (6)		
CHARACTERISTIC	Percent yes	Percent no	TOTAL PERCENT
Age (1)			
1-5	52	48	100
6-17	55	45	100
18-34	49	51	100
35-54	56	44	100
55-64	72	28	100
65 and over	78	22	100
Sex (2)			
Male	54	46	100
Female	61	39	100
Race (3)			
White	63	37	100
Nonwhite	35	65	100
Residence (4)			
SMSA, central city	46	54	100
SMSA, other urban	50	50	100
Urban, non-SMSA	78	22	100
Rural, nonfarm	57	43	100
Rural farm	84	16	100
Poverty level (5)			
Above	63	37	100
Below	46	54	100
Total	57	43	100[a]

[a]Percent table N is of U.S. population equals 18; percent who do not have clinic as regular source of care or NA equals 82.

Respondents who reported having a regular source of care were asked how long it usually took them to get there. An alternative approach to eliciting information about travel time is to query the respondent about how long it took him to get to the doctor's office or other location for his most recent visit with a physician — regardless of whether it was his regular source of care. The 1969 Health Interview Survey, conducted by the National Center for Health Statistics, for example, showed that, for all those who reported a recent visit to a physician, 49.7 percent required fewer than 15 minutes traveling time (NCHS — #10, 1972g).

FINDINGS

The 1970 CHAS survey data, similarly, showed that approximately 50 percent of those with a regular source of care could reach it in less than fifteen minutes (See Table 3).

Older people were less apt to have brief travel times to their regular source of care than were the young. A larger proportion of the older adults and elderly who had a regular source of care had to travel more than half an hour to reach that source.

The travel time required to obtain care did not differ for men and women.

A larger percentage of whites than nonwhites could reach their regular source of care in less than fifteen minutes.

Rural farm residents were much less likely than urban dwellers or rural nonfarm residents to reach their regular source of care in less than fifteen minutes. A larger percentage of the rural farm residents, than the other rural or urban residents, had to travel more than thirty minutes to obtain care.

The nonpoor reported shorter travel times to their regular source of care than did the poor. In the 1969 NCHS study, also, the average traveling time associated with the most recent physician visit was less in families with higher incomes (NCHS — #10, 1972g).

People who reported clinics as their usual source of care had to travel longer to reach them than those who said they had a physician as their regular source of care. The 1969 NCHS survey, too, showed that those persons whose most recent physician visit occurred at a hospital clinic averaged longer travel times (24.4 minutes) than those who visited a physician at his office (17.2 minutes) (NCHS — #10, 1972g).

APPOINTMENT OR WALK-IN VISIT

Having an appointment to obtain services connotes somewhat greater continuity of care than simply walking in to obtain services when the

TABLE 3
Travel time to regular source of care by selected characteristics of population-at-risk

CHARACTERISTIC	TRAVEL TIME (7)				
	Percent less than 15 minutes	Percent 15 to 30 minutes	Percent 31 to 60 minutes	Percent more than one hour	TOTAL PERCENT
Age (1)					
1-5	51	39	9	1	100
6-17	51	41	7	1	100
18-34	52	37	9	2	100
35-54	55	35	8	2	100
55-64	47	40	11	3	101[a]
65 and over	47	38	13	3	101[a]
Sex (2)					
Male	52	38	9	2	101[a]
Female	51	39	9	2	101[a]
Race (3)					
White	54	37	8	2	101[a]
Nonwhite	35	46	16	4	101[a]
Residence (4)					
SMSA, central city	51	40	8	2	101[a]
SMSA, other urban	58	34	7	1	100
Urban, non-SMSA	70	23	6	2	101[a]
Rural, nonfarm	44	44	10	2	100
Rural farm	21	54	21	4	100
Poverty level (5)					
Above	54	38	7	1	100
Below	42	39	16	4	101[a]
Regular source of care (6)					
Clinic	42	41	12	4	99[a]
GP	55	37	7	1	100
Specialist	52	37	10	2	101[a]
Total	51	38	9	2	100[b]

[a]Does not add up to 100 because of rounding error.
[b]Percent table N is of U.S. population equals 87; percent who do not have a regular source of care or NA equals 13.

need arises. People who just walk in to see a doctor may also have a wait longer than those who have scheduled an appointment in advance.

VARIABLE DESCRIPTION

People with a regular source of care were asked whether they usually had an appointment to see their doctor or simply walked in.

FINDINGS

Approximately 75 percent of the people with a regular source of care generally had appointments to see their doctor (See Table 4).

Young children were more apt than the other age groups to have appointments.

There was no difference between males and females with respect to making appointments when they went to see their regular source of care.

Whites were much more apt to have an appointment with their regular care source than nonwhites.

Rural farm residents were more likely to simply walk in to obtain services when the need arose than were rural nonfarm or urban residents.

The nonpoor made appointments to see their regular care source more often than did the poor.

People who see specialists as their regular source of care were more apt to make appointments than those who had clinics or general practitioners as their usual source of care.

APPOINTMENT WAITING TIME

Those persons who want to make appointments to see their physicians often must wait several days before they can be scheduled. This inconvenience undoubtedly contributes to potential consumers' complaints about the medical care system and to expressions of generalized dissatisfaction with the process of care-seeking. It may also reduce demand for service.

VARIABLE DESCRIPTION

People who generally have an appointment to see their regular source of care were asked how long it usually took them to get an appointment.

FINDINGS

Over one-third of those who generally had appointments had to wait three days or longer to be scheduled (See Table 5).

Older adults 55 to 64 years of age were less apt than the other age groups to be able to see the doctor within two days after contacting him for an appointment. The comparatively large percent of children who had to wait more than two weeks to get an appointment may be a

TABLE 4
Appointment or walk-in visit to regular source of care by selected characteristics
of population-at-risk

| | APPOINTMENT OR WALK-IN VISIT (8) | | |
CHARACTERISTIC	Percent with appointment	Percent with walk-in	TOTAL PERCENT
Age (1)			
1-5	81	19	100
6-17	76	24	100
18-34	75	25	100
35-54	77	23	100
55-64	68	32	100
65 and over	76	24	100
Sex (2)			
Male	76	24	100
Female	76	24	100
Race (3)			
White	78	22	100
Nonwhite	60	40	100
Residence (4)			
SMSA, central city	74	26	100
SMSA, other urban	85	15	100
Urban, non-SMSA	77	23	100
Rural nonfarm	71	29	100
Rural farm	59	41	100
Poverty level (5)			
Above	79	21	100
Below	63	37	100
Regular source of care (6)			
Clinic	71	29	100
GP	71	29	100
Specialist	90	11	101[a]
Total	76	24	100[b]

[a]Does not add up to 100 because of rounding error.

[b]Percent table N is of U.S. population equals 87; percent who do not have a regular source of care or NA equals 13.

TABLE 5
Appointment waiting time at regular source of care by selected characteristics of population-at-risk

| | APPOINTMENT WAITING TIME (9) | | | |
| | Percent same day to 2 days | Percent 3 days to 2 weeks | Percent more than 2 weeks | TOTAL PERCENT |
CHARACTERISTIC				
Age (1)				
1-5	64	24	12	100
6-17	64	29	8	101[a]
18-34	62	29	9	100
35-54	63	30	8	101[a]
55-64	58	32	10	100
65 and over	62	29	9	100
Sex (2)				
Male	65	27	8	100
Female	60	30	10	100
Race (3)				
White	62	29	9	100
Nonwhite	64	26	10	100
Residence (4)				
SMSA, central city	54	33	14	101[a]
SMSA, other urban	66	26	9	101[a]
Urban, non-SMSA	68	29	3	100
Rural nonfarm	65	28	7	100
Rural farm	68	26	7	101[a]
Poverty level (5)				
Above	63	28	9	101[a]
Below	63	31	6	100
Regular source of care (6)				
Clinic	55	34	12	101[a]
GP	69	24	6	99[a]
Specialist	55	33	12	100
Total	63	29	9	101[a,b]

[a]Does not add up to 100 because of rounding error.

[b]Percent table N is of U.S. population equals 65; percent who do not have a regular source of care, or who have a regular source but do not usually have an appointment with him, or NA equals 35.

function of the kinds of care they receive (periodic preventive checkups) and the fact that they were more apt to see specialists.

Males were somewhat more likely than females to get an appointment to see the doctor within a couple of days of requesting it.

There was little difference in the appointment waiting times between whites and nonwhites.

People who live in the SMSA inner cities had longer waits to get an appointment with their doctor than did people living in other parts of the city or in rural areas.

The percent waiting more than two weeks to get an appointment was somewhat higher for the nonpoor than the poor.

People who have general practitioners as their regular source of care were more apt to get an appointment in a couple of days than were those persons who reported clinics or specialists as their regular care source.

OFFICE WAITING TIME

People complain that they must often wait long periods of time in a doctor's office before being seen. These long waiting times are apt to influence where people choose to go for care, how often they go, and how satisfied they are with the care they eventually receive.

VARIABLE DESCRIPTION

People with a regular source of care were asked how long they usually had to wait to see the doctor, once they were in his office.

FINDINGS

Twenty percent of those who reported a regular source of care had to wait more than an hour to see their doctor (See Table 6).

Older adults and children 6-17 were more likely to have waits of 30 minutes or more to see a physician than the other age groups.

Men were somewhat more apt to see the doctor immediately or within half an hour than women.

Nonwhites generally had much longer waits in a doctor's office than did white patients.

Rural farm residents were apt to report the longest waits to see a physician and SMSA residents outside the inner-city were more likely to see the doctor within thirty minutes than people in the other residence categories.

The poor (many of whom are nonwhite, also) report long waiting times before seeing a physician. The nonpoor were more apt than the poor to see a doctor immediately.

People who reported specialists as their regular source of care were more likely to see the doctor immediately than people who went to

TABLE 6
Office waiting time at regular source of care by selected characteristics of
population-at-risk

CHARACTERISTIC	OFFICE WAITING TIME (10)				
	Percent immediate	Percent 1 to 30 minutes	Percent 31 to 60 minutes	Percent more than one hour	TOTAL PERCENT
Age (1)					
1-5	8	52	22	18	100
6-17	6	48	25	22	101[a]
18-34	7	53	23	18	101[a]
35-54	7	49	27	17	100
55-64	9	43	23	24	99[a]
65 and over	6	47	26	22	101[a]
Sex (2)					
Male	7	50	24	19	100
Female	6	48	25	20	99[a]
Race (3)					
White	7	51	24	18	100
Nonwhite	3	36	28	33	100
Residence (4)					
SMSA, central city	8	47	21	25	101[a]
SMSA, other urban	7	58	24	11	100
Urban, non-SMSA	6	49	27	18	100
Rural nonfarm	7	47	24	22	100
Rural farm	4	29	39	28	100
Poverty level (5)					
Above	8	53	24	16	101[a]
Below	4	36	27	33	100
Regular source of care (6)					
Clinic	5	44	24	26	99[a]
GP	7	46	25	23	101[a]
Specialist	9	57	24	10	100
Total	7	49	24	20	100[b]

[a]Does not add up to 100 because of rounding error.
[b]Percent table N is of U.S. population equals 87; percent who do not have a regular source of care or NA equals 13.

clinics or general practitioners. Clinic users reported the longest waiting times before seeing a docotor.

The time that one must wait to see a physician is undoubtedly influenced by whether or not one has an appointment to see him. The 1969 NCHS Health Interview Survey showed that 43.8 percent of patients with an appointment waited less than 15 minutes to see the physician in his office, compared to 37.6 percent of the people with *no* appointment (NCHS — #10, 1972g).

Table 7 shows that, according to the 1970 CHAS survey data, people who generally had appointments with their regular source of care were more apt to see him immediately or within thirty minutes than were those who simply walked in for a visit. This relationship is true, in general, for all of the population subgroups being studied.

SUMMARY AND EVALUATION OF PROCESS INDICES

The preceding analyses have suggested that, based on selected process indices, some groups have better access to the medical care system than others (See Table 8). Children, in general, have more of an advantage with respect to having a usual source of care that is convenient to them than do adults. Older adults, 55 to 64 years of age, and the elderly, must often travel more than an hour to reach care. The 55 to 64 year-olds are also more likely to have unscheduled visits to a physician. Once in the doctor's office, they also have the longest waits.

Men are more likely than women to have no usual source of care, but they have shorter waits to get an appointment or see the doctor, once in his office, than do women.

Nonwhites less often have a usual source of care than do whites. Their care is usually less convenient — based on travel time, whether it is a walk-in visit or not, appointment waiting time, and the time spent in the physician's office waiting to be seen.

Residents of the inner-city and rural farm dwellers are the most disadvantaged with respect to having a regular source of care that is conveniently available to them.

People below the poverty level are more likely to have no regular source of care, to have to travel more than thirty minutes to obtain services, to have walk-in visits and to wait more than thirty minutes in the doctor's office before seeing him than are the nonpoor.

Those who identify clinics as their usual care source generally have less convenient care than people who report a medical doctor as their usual care source. People who go to general practitioners, as do clinic users, are more apt to simply walk-in to obtain care than are those who use specialists. People who make appointments to see specialists generally have longer waits before being scheduled than do those who go to general practitioners.

These findings suggest that the process indices of access introduced here may be of value in discriminating subgroups that have less access to medical care. There are formal criteria that may be applied to further appraise the overall usefulness of these measures as access indicators, however — with respect to their validity, reliability, variance, ease of collection, ease of computation, ease of interpretation and mutability.

Validity refers to the extent to which differences in the index reflect true differences in access for the people for whom the data are collected. Face validity refers to whether the measure "makes sense" as an indicator of the access concept. Content validity means whether the item is a sample from the universe in which the investigator is interested. Predictive validity is a reference to the capacity of a measure for predicting some outcome score.

All of the indicators introduced here seem to fare well on these different validity criteria. Whether or not one has a regular source of medical care and the ease of convenience of getting there all seem to "make sense" as indicators of the population's access to the system. These measures sample the universe of items with which researchers have traditionally been concerned in describing access to medical care. The existing literature on these different indicators suggest that they are predictive of the site, contact, volume and continuity of care-seeking and the consumers' satisfaction with it. In the preliminary analyses of the outcome indices that follow, more attention will be directed to evaluating how use patterns and satisfaction vary for some of these indices — to provide a more direct test of their predictive capacity.

Reliability refers to the consistency of independent, but comparable measures over time (stability) and situations (equivalence).

No direct assessment of the reliability of these measures is undertaken here. However, previous studies have asked similar questions with respect to the population's usual source of care and similar distributions of people with no regular source and doctors or clinics as their usual source of care, by poverty level and race, for example, were found (Bice, 1971; Donabedian and Rosenfeld, 1961; Richardson, 1970).

The variance of an index means that there should be some variability in the measure, to detect true differences over time and place. This criterion is somewhat a composite of the validity and reliability criteria. We would expect a social indicator of access to vary over time and place as a function of true differences in access. The variability should, however, result from underlying substantive differences, rather than the idiosyncracies (or unreliability) of the index.

TABLE 7
Office waiting time at regular source of care by appointment or walk-in visit by selected characteristics of population-at-risk

	OFFICE WAITING TIME (10)[a]							
	Percent immediate		Percent 1 to 30 minutes		Percent 31 to 60 minutes		Percent more than one hour	
	APPOINTMENT OR WALK-IN VISIT (8)							
CHARACTERISTIC	Appointment	Walk-in	Appointment	Walk-in	Appointment	Walk-in	Appointment	Walk-in
Age (1)								
Under 65	8	4	55	32	22	32	16	31
65 and over	6	6	55	23	25	28	15	43
Sex (2)								
Male	8	5	56	33	21	31	15	31
Female	7	4	54	30	23	32	16	34
Race (3)								
White	8	5	56	33	22	32	15	30
Nonwhite	3	2	44	24	27	29	26	44
Residence (4)								
Urban	7	5	56	35	22	30	15	31
Rural	7	5	51	26	24	34	18	35
Poverty level (5)								
Above	8	6	57	36	21	33	14	25
Below	5	3	45	22	26	28	24	48
Regular source of care (6)								
Clinic	5	5	51	26	22	30	21	39
GP	8	3	53	30	22	33	18	34
Specialist	8	13	68	46	24	23	10	18
Total[b]	7	5	55	31	22	32	16	33

[a]In this table percentages are computed so that in any row the sum across a particular appointment or walk-in visit category equals 100, subject to rounding error. For example, in the first row for Appointment, Age under 65: 8+55+22+16=101.
[b]Percent table N is of U.S. population equals 86; percent who do not have a regular source of care or NA equals 14.

The findings reported for the indices for selected characteristics of the population-at-risk suggest that there is meaningful variance in these measures for the different age, sex, race, etc. categories.

Policy makers and others who want to evaluate access are apt to favor those indices for which data may be easily collected. The data on the process indices just examined can be easily collected, through questions that have been pre-tested and included on a variety of national and local studies. In contrast to the approach used in the last CHAS study, the travel time, appointment waiting time, etc. may be asked with respect to the most recent contact with the medical system, instead of the usual source of care — as in the 1969 NCHS study. Collecting the data in this way may offer some advantages in terms of the reliability and generalizability of the findings. Asking these questions in terms of the most recent contact provides a more concrete reference point in time for the respondent. Further, information can be collected for all those who had a contact with a physician in the given time period, regardless of whether they have a regular source of care or not.

As reported here, the findings on the respective indices are relatively straightforward and easily computed. One may, as Chen (1973) did in his preliminary model of access combine some of the travel and waiting time indices into a single summary score.

Another attribute of a good index of access to medical care, however, is that it be easily interpreted. Administrators and policy makers must be able to translate the indices developed into concrete decisions and policy.

This disadvantage of developing a composite index of travel and waiting time, etc. as Chen suggests, may be that it is not as easily interpretable, nor as easily translated into decisions about how care should be re-organized, as the different dimensions considered separately would be.

Mutability refers to how manipulable the underlying conditions reflected in the index are by health policy. If the factors the indices reflect are ones that policy makers can do little to change, then perhaps they are of less interest as direct "social indicators" of access.

The process indices reported here — regular source of care, travel time, appointment or walk-in visit, appointment and office waiting time — do, in general, reflect aspects of the medical care system that policy makers may seek to alter — to improve access to care.

TABLE 8
Summary of population groups with "least access"[a] according to process indicators

CHARACTERISTIC	No Regular Source of Care (6)	Travel Time More Than One Hour (7)	Walk-In Visit (8)	Appointment Waiting Time More Than Two Weeks (9)	Office Waiting Time More Than One Hour (10)
Age (1)	Adults 18-54	Adults 55 and over	Adults 55-64	Children 1-5	Adults 55-64
Sex (2)	Males	No Difference	No difference	Females	Females
Race (3)	Nonwhites	Nonwhites	Nonwhites	No difference	Nonwhites
Residence (4)	SMSA, central city	Rural farm	Rural farm	SMSA, central city	Rural farm
Poverty level (5)	Below	Below	Below	Above	Below
Regular source of care (6)	—	Clinic	Clinic and GP	Clinic and specialist	Clinic

[a]The groups with the "least access" are based on which subcategories of the characteristics of the population-at-risk had the highest proportions in the extreme categories of the process indicators reported here.

Outcome Indices of Access

As discussed in the theoretical review of the access concept, utilization and satisfaction indices may serve as outcome indicators of individuals' entry to and passage through the medical care system.

In the sections that follow, selected outcome indicators of access are introduced, findings on them from secondary analyses of the 1970 CHAS survey are reported, and the relative advantage and disadvantage of each is evaluated.

Four main types of outcome indices will be reviewed: (1) conventional utilization measures; (2) measures of the use of services relative to the need for services; (3) continuity of care indices; and (4) satisfaction with care scales. They will be analyzed and compared for the same population subgroup reported for the process indexes.

CONVENTIONAL USE MEASURES

Percent (Not) Seeing a Physician

An important measure of the use of services that has appeared frequently in the literature is the percentage of the population who see a physician during the year. It is probably the clearest measure of gross exposure of the public to a physician's decisions. Obviously, the physician cannot prescribe care until he talks with or sees a patient.

In terms of access, then, policy makers may be especially concerned with those groups in which a large percentage of the members have *no* contact with the medical care system in the year. The percent *not* seeing a physician is probably an intuitively more interesting statistic to report to evaluate access, then, than is the percent who do.

VARIABLE DESCRIPTION

The proportion of people who were in the population during all twelve months of 1970 (excluded are people who were born and died or who were institutionalized or left the country during the year) that had at least one visit to a physician constitute the "percent seeing a physician in 1970." The remainder is, of course, the percent who did not.

FINDINGS

In 1970, according to the CHAS survey of that year, almost a third of the United States population did not see a physician (See Table 9).

Children 6 to 17 were more apt than the other age groups to have had no contact with a physician during the survey year.

Men, more so than women, were more likely not to have seen the physician.

TABLE 9

Percent (not) seeing a physician in 1970 by selected characteristics of population-at-risk

| | PERCENT SEEING A PHYSICIAN (11) | | TOTAL |
CHARACTERISTIC	Yes	No	PERCENT
Age (1)			
1-5	75	25	100
6-17	62	38	100
18-34	70	30	100
35-54	67	33	100
55-64	73	27	100
65 and over	76	24	100
Sex (2)			
Male	65	35	100
Female	71	29	100
Race (3)			
White	70	30	100
Nonwhite	58	42	100
Residence (4)			
SMSA, central city	65	35	100
SMSA, other urban	72	28	100
Urban, non-SMSA	71	29	100
Rural nonfarm	68	32	100
Rural farm	62	38	100
Poverty level (5)			
Above	71	29	100
Below	58	42	100
Regular source of care (6)			
None	36	64	100
Clinic	70	30	100
GP	68	32	100
Specialist	82	18	100
Total	68	32	100[a]

[a]Percent table N is of U.S. population equals 97; percent who were not in universe all twelve months of 1970 equals 3.

The percentage of nonwhites not seeing the doctor was higher than the percentage of whites.

Rural farm residents were least apt to have had a contact with a physician in the survey year and SMSA residents outside the central city most likely to see a doctor.

A substantially larger proportion of the poor (42%) than the nonpoor (29%) did not see a doctor in 1970. The percent of the poor not seeing a doctor was much higher than the national average (32%).

People who had no regular source of care were twice as likely not to have seen a doctor in the survey year as those who had a doctor as their usual source of care. The proportion not seeing a doctor was least for those who reported a specialist as their usual source of care. It should be remembered, however, that those who have had occasion to see a physician during the year may be more inclined to report a regular source of care than are people who did not receive physician care.

Mean Number of Physician Visits

The mean number of physician visits is a frequently cited volume measure of health service use. It incorporates both the number of initial contacts and return visits to a physician. The return visits, more so than the initial contacts with the provider, are influenced by how the system is organized with respect to provider decision-making referral patterns, etc.

VARIABLE DESCRIPTION

The mean number of physician visits overall and for those who had one or more visits is reported in Table 10 (See Chapter 3 for more detailed description of what kinds of visits were included). The overall mean includes those who had no contact with the system in the year. The second mean is computed only for those who saw a physician at least once during the survey year.

FINDINGS

In 1970 there were, on the average, four visits to a physician per person overall nationally (including those who did not see a doctor at all). Those who saw a physician at least once, however, averaged almost six visits per person (see Table 10).

Children 6 to 17 averaged fewest visits to the physician. Older adults and the elderly had the most visits overall.

Males generally averaged fewer visits to the doctor than females. The gap narrowed somewhat, when considering only those who got into the system. Females continued to average slightly more visits than males, however.

The mean number of physician visits overall was less for nonwhites

TABLE 10
Mean number of physician visits per person-year overall and for those with one
or more visits by selected characteristics of population-at-risk

| | MEAN NUMBER OF PHYSICIAN VISITS (12) | |
CHARACTERISTIC	Overall	One or more visits
Age (1)		
1-5	3.5	4.8
6-17	2.2	3.6
18-34	4.2	6.1
35-54	4.0	6.0
55-64	6.3	9.0
65 and over	6.4	8.7
Sex (2)		
Male	3.6	5.6
Female	4.5	6.3
Race (3)		
White	4.1	5.9
Nonwhite	3.6	6.2
Residence (4)		
SMSA, central city	4.2	6.5
SMSA, other urban	4.2	5.8
Urban, non-SMSA	4.4	6.3
Rural nonfarm	3.7	5.5
Rural farm	3.4	5.6
Poverty level (5)		
Above	4.0	5.7
Below	4.0	6.9
Regular source of care (6)		
None	1.3	3.5
Clinic	4.0	5.9
GP	3.8	5.6
Specialist	5.6	7.0
Total	4.0	5.9

than whites. Once in the system, however, the nonwhites averaged slightly more visits than the whites. This finding and the previous table on the percent (not) seeing a physician suggest that though nonwhites may delay longer before seeing a physician than whites, once in the system, they require more visits to get their health problem resolved.

Rural farm and nonfarm dwellers averaged fewer visits to a physician than city residents, overall. Once they see a doctor, the relative difference between the rural and urban residents becomes less. SMSA inner-city residents, however, average the most visits to physicians, once in the system.

The mean number of physician visits for the poor and nonpoor were identical in 1970 overall. This convergence suggests that programs directed specifically at improving access to the medical care for the poor (Medicaid, Medicare, etc.) may have met with some success. When considering only those who got into the system, the poor, in fact, averaged more visits to a physician than the nonpoor. As with the white-nonwhite distinction, though the poor wait longer to see a doctor, once in the system, they require more care than those with higher incomes.

People who had no regular source of care averaged the fewest visits to a physician in 1970 and those who reported a specialist as their usual source of care, the most. The relative difference in use narrows somewhat once a physician is contacted, but those with no regular source of care continue to average the least and those with a specialist as their regular source of care the most visits to a physician, once in the system.

In general, these findings affirm that some groups (especially nonwhites, central city and rural residents, the poor and those with no regular source of care) delay longer in seeking the services of a physician. By the time they do see a doctor, however, the severity of their condition has probably increased, so that more visits to a physician are required to remedy it. For some groups, then, who have low rates of initial "contact" with the system — nonwhites and the poor, for example — compared to others, once in the system they averaged more visits to a doctor than their (white and nonpoor) counterparts.

Some of the groups found to have less access to care, based on these conventional use indices, were also the people found to be at a disadvantage with respect to the process indicators of access. In subsequent analyses, other outcome-type access indicators will be examined to see how these same population subgroups fare — and to see what additional information might be provided on the "process and behavioral and subjective outcomes of individuals' entry to the medical care system" by such measures.

NEED-BASED USE MEASURES

Access to medical care is perhaps best considered in the context of whether people who need care receive it. At present, however, there is a dearth of indices that permit the use of services relative to the need for services to be measured. Morbidity data are collected for different groups, independent of their use of physician services. Similarly, the volume of physician service use is reported with no indication of the groups' need for care. In the analyses that follow, some of the conventional "contact" and "volume" indices of use just reviewed will be analyzed in the context of peoples' actual *need* for medical services. Such measures provide a more direct test of whether people who really need care receive it or not.

As mentioned in the theoretical discussion of the access concept, medical need may be either perceived by the individual or evaluated by health care professionals. The need-based use measures to be introduced here, incorporate indices of both perceived (disability days, symptoms) and medically-evaluated (symptom severity and medical condition severity) need. In some of the indices, the medically-determined need measures are used as normative criteria, against which the "appropriateness" of patients' responses to perceived morbidity are evaluated.

Use-Disability Ratio

The use-disability ratio introduced by the National Center for Health Services Research and Development (now the Bureau of Health Services Research and Evaluation) is one attempt to develop an index of access to medical care that integrates the rates of use and need in a population into a single measure, so that the discrepancy between need in a population and seeking physician services in response to it can be computed. The ratio basically consists of the number of physician visits in two weeks per 100 disability (bed and restricted activity) days in two weeks.

According to the designers of the ratio:

> The use-need discrepancy ratio[2], . . . as an *index of access to health services,* deviates from the traditional approach to using utilization of services alone. Since the use of health services is highly related to the prevalence of illness, differences in amount of utilization may simply reflect different levels of health, not access.

---

[2]The National Center for Health Services Research and Development (NCHSRD) termed this particular index a "use-need discrepancy ratio." We have called it the "use-*disability* ratio," to better distinguish the criterion of medical need employed in constructing it.

Therefore, a more appropriate index of access is the ratio (or discrepancy) of use to need for services, indicated by disability days. This discrepancy, in turn, can be related to characteristics of the population such as income, race, and place of residence (Health Services Research and Training Program, 1972:6).

VARIABLE DESCRIPTION

The computational formula for the use-disability ratio is as follows:

$$(1)\ \text{use-disability ratio} = \frac{\displaystyle\frac{\sum_{i=1}^{n} MD_i}{n}}{\displaystyle\frac{\sum_{i=1}^{n} DD_i}{n}}(100) = \frac{\text{mean } MD_i}{\text{mean } DD_i}(100), \text{ where}$$

MD_i =   number of physician visits in two weeks made by an individual i who had at least one disability day in two weeks

DD_i =   number of disability days in two weeks for an individual i who had at least one disability day in two weeks.

FINDINGS

Table 11 provides some preliminary data on whether people who experienced disability in the two-week reporting period saw a physician or not. Tables 12-14 provide data on the use-disability ratio itself, which looks at the *volume* of physician use relative to the number of days of limited activity people in the sample experienced.

Slightly more than 60 percent of the people who had disability days in the two-week period did not contact a doctor in response to them (See Table 11). The majority of people, then, who had to take time out from their normal routine in the past few weeks due to illness did not bother to see the doctor about it.

In general, the population subgroups who were apt not to have seen the doctor at all during the year — children 6-17, males, rural farm residents, the poor and the people with no regular source of care (Table 9) — did not see the doctor, even when ill health interrupted their normal

TABLE 11
Percent with disability days in two weeks who had one or more physician visits in two weeks by selected characteristics of population-at-risk

| | PERCENT WITH DISABILITY DAYS WHO SAW DOCTOR (13,14) | | TOTAL PERCENT |
CHARACTERISTIC	Yes	No	
Age (1)			
1-5	50	50	100
6-17	34	67	101[a]
18-34	39	62	101[a]
35-54	50	51	101[a]
55-64	33	67	100
65 and over	41	59	100
Sex (2)			
Male	39	61	100
Female	41	59	100
Race (3)			
White	40	60	100
Nonwhite	36	64	100
Residence (4)			
SMSA, central city	40	60	100
SMSA, other urban	40	60	100
Urban, non-SMSA	42	58	100
Rural nonfarm	40	60	100
Rural farm	38	62	100
Property level (5)			
Above	42	58	100
Below	34	66	100
Regular source of care (6)			
None	26	74	100
Clinic	43	57	100
GP	34	66	100
Specialist	51	50	101[a]
Total	39	61	100[b]

[a]Does not add up to 100 because of rounding error.

[b]Percent table N is of U.S. population equals 17; percent who did not have at least one disability day in two weeks or NA equals 83.

routine or forced them to stay in bed. The differences in the percentage of the different age, sex, race, etc. subgroups who did not see a doctor was, however, much less among those who experienced a disabling health problem recently. The percent of males and females with disability who did not see a doctor was, for example, quite similar (61 and 59, respectively). When considering only those who experienced disability days, people in the age group 55-64 did, however, appear not to contact a doctor as often as those in some of the other age categories.

Looking at the use-disability ratio itself (Table 12), for every 100 days of limited activity in the population, there were approximately 14 visits to a physician.

Analysis of the use-disability ratio by age shows that the use of services relative to the need for services is lowest for older adults, age 55-64 (7.64); highest for adults in the middle years 35-54 (18.73) and very young children (17.95); and moderate (14.11) for the elderly. Mean disability days increase with age. Mean physician visits, however, are highest for adults 65 and over (1.24).

Though the elderly average more physician visits than any other age group, their use of services relative to need is moderate, compared to the other age categories. Older adults, ages 55-64, have very low rates of use, relative to the days of disability they experience. These older adults like the elderly, report high levels of need. Unlike the people 65 and over, however, they are not covered by Medicare. This factor may account for why they are less apt to see a doctor when the need arises than the elderly. Adults in the middle years, 35-54, comprise the bulk of the employed working force. They are apt to have the benefits of employer-subsidized health insurance and company- or industry-owned clinics, so that when the need arises, there are fewer barriers to their obtaining medical services. The higher score on the use-need discrepancy ratio for children one to five years of age is probably due to their greater use of preventive services and the tendency of parents to contact a doctor by phone regarding the child's health.

Physician visits per 100 disability days are quite similar for men (14.12) and women (14.78). Women experience slightly more disability, but they also average more physician visits than men.

Women are more apt to experience disability days than men, because of debilitating periods during pregnancy. They also see a doctor more often than men. Relative to their respective need for care then, men and women use services at very similar rates — as reflected in the use-disability ratio.

The use-disability ratio is higher for whites (14.84) than nonwhites (12.88). Whites average the most physician visits, but nonwhites report the most disability.

TABLE 12
Physician visits in two weeks per 100 disability days in two weeks, mean
physician visits and mean disability days for those with one or more disability
days by selected characteristics of population-at-risk

CHARACTERISTIC	USE-DISABILITY RATIO	MEAN PHYSICIAN VISITS FOR THOSE WITH ONE OR MORE DISABILITY DAYS (14)	MEAN DISABILITY DAYS FOR THOSE WITH ONE OR MORE DISABILITY DAYS (13)
Age (1)			
1-5	17.95	.79	4.40
6-17	12.78	.52	4.07
18-34	16.59	.70	4.22
35-54	18.73	1.06	5.66
55-64	7.64	.62	8.12
65 and over	14.11	1.24	8.79
Sex (2)			
Male	14.12	.75	5.31
Female	14.78	.81	5.48
Race (3)			
White	14.84	.80	5.39
Nonwhite	12.88	.72	5.59
Residence (4)			
SMSA, central city	15.29	.85	5.56
SMSA, other urban	15.66	.83	5.30
Urban, non-SMSA	14.70	.71	4.83
Rural nonfarm	12.52	.69	5.51
Rural farm	12.26	.71	5.79
Poverty level (5)			
Above	16.37	.82	5.01
Below	10.37	.68	6.56
Regular source of care (6)			
None	10.46	.52	4.97
Clinic	16.67	.94	5.64
GP	12.94	.66	5.10
Specialist	16.69	.99	5.93
Total[a]	14.41	.78	5.41

[a]Percent table N is of U.S. population equals 17; percent who did not have one or more disability
days in two weeks, NA equals 83.

Whites, then, are somewhat more apt than nonwhites to see a doctor when the need arises. Controlling the relationship of race to the use-need discrepancy ratio for income (which will be done later in this analysis) permits a test of whether this difference is primarily due to economic factors.

Rural farm residents report the fewest physician visits per 100 days of disability experienced (12.26) and non-inner city residents of Standard Metropolitan Statistical Areas (SMSA's), the most physician visits per 100 disability days (15.66). Rural residents experience the highest rates of disability, but city dwellers average the most visits to a doctor.

Rural farm dwellers are apt to be older and of lower socio-economic status than the suburbanites represented in the high-scoring "SMSA, other urban" category.

The poor average more disability days (6.56) than the nonpoor (5.01). Mean physician visits are slightly lower for the poor (.68) than the nonpoor (.82). Physician visits per 100 disability days are, therefore, less for the poor (10.37) than the nonpoor (16.37).

Table 10 showed that, overall, the poor and nonpoor appeared to be seeing a physician at similar rates. Once in the system the poor, in fact, saw the doctor more often than the more well-to-do. The use-disability ratio, however, shows that relative to their actual need for care, the poor may continue to use fewer services than the nonpoor.

People who had specialists as their regular source of care averaged the most disability days in two weeks (5.93), but they also had the most physician visits (.99). The fewest visits were reported by those who had no regular place they went for medical advice and treatment. The use of services relative to need, using the use-disability ratio, was least for those who had no regular source of care (10.46) and highest for those with specialists (16.69) or clinics (16.67) as their regular source of care.

To explore the factors that may be contributing to the differences in the use-disability ratio for the different groups, in more detail, Table 13 summarizes a rank-ordering of the ratio (high to low) for a cross-classification of selected income, residence, race and age categories.

These findings affirm that people above the poverty level consistently have higher scores on the index (more physician visits relative to need) than do those below the poverty level. For the nonpoor — urban dwellers generally have higher rates of access to needed medical care than do the residents of rural areas. The groups which have the highest values on the index are the nonpoor, urban whites. These people are probably middle- and upper-class city residents, insured through Medicare and other third-party payers. Poor elderly nonwhites concentrated in the central city have the lowest rates of use relative to their actual need for care (3.55). And the elderly, rural poor — of both races — have much lower rates of use relative to their need for care than do the younger rural poor or the nonpoor urban dwellers.

People who report large numbers of disability days are undoubtedly of special interest to policy makers and others concerned with whether the people who really need care get it or not. Subsequently, Table 14 summarizes the findings on the use-disability ratio for people who experienced six or more days of limited activity during the two-week reporting period.

In general, the use-disability ratio is lower for this group, suggesting that the number of physician visits relative to the number of days of disability experienced is less for those who report a larger number of limited-activity days.

Those population subgroups which had the lowest rates of use relative to need in the more general analyses of the use-disability ratio also have the lowest rates of use relative to need, when those who experienced large numbers of disability days, only, are considered. Adults 55-64, nonwhites, rural farm dwellers, the poor and those with no regular source of care continued to have the lowest scores on the use-disability ratio. The more generalized ratio, then does seem to reflect relative differences in access for those people *most* in need of care.

Symptoms-Response Ratio[3]

A second need-based use measure that may be of interest in evaluating the use of services relative to the need for services is the symptoms-response ratio. This index is based on the discrepancy between the actual number of visits to a physician for a given mix of symptoms and estimates from a panel of medical professional experts of the number of visits that should occur for these symptoms. Unlike the use-disability ratio, the symptoms-response index incorporates an explicit external norm of medical appropriateness, against which the population's actual responses to perceived symptoms of illness may be compared.

VARIABLE DESCRIPTION

The symptoms-response ratio makes use of a checklist of symptoms administered to all persons or their proxies over one year of age in the 1970 Center for Health Administration Studies nationwide survey. For each of the 22 symptoms on the list, people were asked whether or not they experienced the symptom during the survey year and, if the symptom was reported, whether or not a doctor was seen about it.

---

[3]The physician rankings used in this ratio were collected by Ronald Klar, M.D. and much of the computational development was provided by D. Garth Taylor.

TABLE 13
Physician visits in two weeks per 100 disability days in two weeks by poverty
level by residence by race by age

CHARACTERISTIC[a]	USE-DISABILITY RATIO
Above poverty level, urban, white, 65 and over	21.32
urban, white, under 65	16.84
urban, nonwhite, under 65	15.45
rural, white, 65 and over	15.19
rural, white, under 65	14.08
Below poverty level, urban, nonwhite, under 65	13.07
urban, white, 65 and over	11.80
rural, white, under 65	11.03
rural, nonwhite, under 65	10.13
urban, white, under 65	9.83
rural, nonwhite, 65 and over	8.04
rural, white, 65 and over	7.15
urban, nonwhite, 65 and over	3.55

[a]The unweighted N for the following categories was less than or equal to 25 and, hence, are not reported: above poverty level, urban, nonwhite, 65 and over; and above poverty level, rural, nonwhite, under 65 *and* 65 and over.

In addition, a panel of forty doctors from the teaching faculty of the University of Chicago School of Medicine were asked to estimate, based on their training and experience, what percentage of the people in a particular age group with that symptom should see a physician for it.

The symptoms-response ratio is based on the difference between the actual number of symptoms for which a visit to the doctor was made and the physician estimates of the number of people with that symptom who should have seen the doctor for that symptom. The computational formula for the index then is, basically, as follows.

(2) symptoms[4]- response ratio $= \dfrac{A - E}{E} (100)$, where

A = actual number of visits for symptoms
E = M.D. estimates of number of visits there "should be" for symptoms

[4]See Chapter 3 for discussion of how the physician estimates were derived and a more detailed discussion of the rationale for this particular computational formula for the symptoms-response ratio.

TABLE 14
Physician visits in two weeks per 100 disability days in two weeks, mean physician visits and mean disability days for those with six or more disability days by selected characteristics of population-at-risk

CHARACTERISTIC	USE-DISABILITY RATIO	MEAN PHYSICIAN VISITS FOR THOSE WITH SIX OR MORE DISABILITY DAYS (14)	MEAN DISABILITY DAYS FOR THOSE WITH SIX OR MORE DISABILITY DAYS (13)
Age (1)			
1-5	13.77	1.19	8.64
6-17	13.41	1.25	9.32
18-34	15.59	1.70	10.90
35-54	17.34	1.93	11.13
55-64	7.21	.88	12.20
65 and over	12.41	1.66	13.37
Sex (2)			
Male	13.16	1.49	11.32
Female	13.72	1.49	10.86
Race (3)			
White	13.58	1.50	11.04
Nonwhite	12.48	1.38	11.05
Residence (4)			
SMSA, central city	14.87	1.80	12.10
SMSA, other urban	14.82	1.58	10.66
Urban, non-SMSA	13.64	1.37	10.04
Rural nonfarm	10.74	1.14	10.61
Rural farm	10.29	1.15	11.17
Poverty level (5)			
Above	15.83	1.71	10.86
Below	9.12	1.04	11.40
Regular source of care (6)			
None	10.36	1.05	10.13
Clinic	13.88	1.54	11.09
GP	12.26	1.39	11.33
Specialist	15.50	1.69	10.90
Total[a]	13.49	1.49	11.04

[a]Percent table N is of U.S. population equals 6; percent who did not have six or more disability days in two weeks, NA equals 94.

This formula reflects the extent to which the actual number of visits in response to a mix of symptoms is greater than, equal to or less than, the number of panel a medical professional experts would recommend.

FINDINGS

Table 15 provides some descriptive data on the distribution of people in each of the population subgroups, with respect to whether they had as many, more, or fewer visits for symptoms than the panel of doctors thought necessary.

Approximately 52 percent of those with symptoms saw the doctor less often than the physicians thought they should, given the medically-significant nature of their reported symptoms. The population subgroups that seemed to consult a physician less often than the doctors estimated they should were adults, nonwhites, rural farm residents, people below the poverty level and particularly those who reported having no regular source of care. The same groups, then, that were found to have less access, based on the process and previously-analyzed outcome indicators of access, also seem to see a doctor less often than a panel of medical professional experts would deem appropriate.

Table 16 provides data on the symptoms-response ratio itself for these groups. The overall ratio for the sample is 0, indicating that, for the general U.S. population, people do not see a physician any more or less often for symptoms than medically-determined norms of appropriateness would suggest they should.

The age groups most apt to have significantly more visits to a doctor than the severity of their symptoms require are children and adolescents (under 18 years of age). Young adults 18-34 saw doctors in response to symptoms at rates similar to those the panel of doctors would recommend. Older adults, especially those 35-64 years of age, went to see a doctor less often when symptoms arose than they should have.

On the use-disability ratio, too, children had high rates of use relative to their need compared to other age groups. Older adults 55-64 had very low rates of use relative to need compared to the other age categories, using the use-disability ratio. The symptoms-response ratio similarly affirms that using symptoms as the criteria of need, there are a large number of people in this age group who do not see a physician as often as they should. The age group 35-54, however, seems to be at somewhat more of an advantage, with respect to seeing a physician when the need arises — using the use-disability ratio — than in the symptoms-response measure. Perhaps this difference is due to the nature of the need criterion in the use-disability ratio. People 35-54, who constitute the bulk of the employed labor force, may be required to contact a doctor to attest

TABLE 15
Percent with symptoms seeing a doctor as often, more often, and less often than physicians estimate they should[a] by selected characteristics of population-at-risk

| | PERCENT WITH SYMPTOMS SEEING A DOCTOR (15,16) | | |
CHARACTERISTIC	Percent seeing doctor as often or more often than they should	Percent seeing doctor less often than they should	TOTAL PERCENT
Age (1)			
1-5	67	33	100
6-17	56	44	100
18-34	45	55	100
35-54	42	58	100
55-64	44	56	100
65 and over	45	55	100
Sex (2)			
Male	47	53	100
Female	49	51	100
Race (3)			
White	48	52	100
Nonwhite	44	56	100
Residence (4)			
SMSA, central city	47	53	100
SMSA, other urban	48	53	101[b]
Urban, non-SMSA	50	50	100
Rural nonfarm	51	49	100
Rural farm	40	60	100
Poverty level (5)			
Above	49	51	100
Below	44	56	100
Regular source of care (6)			
None	20	80	100
Clinic	48	52	100
GP	47	53	100
Specialist	58	42	100
Total	48	52	100[c]

[a]See Chapter 3 for further discussion of how these evaluations of appropriateness are determined for individuals.

[b]Does not add up to 100 because of rounding error.

[c]Percent table N is of U.S. population equals 59; percent who did not experience symptoms or NA equals 41.

TABLE 16
Symptoms-response ratio by selected characteristics of population-at-risk

CHARACTERISTIC	ACTUAL NO. OF VISITS FOR SYMPTOMS (A) (15)[a]	ESTIMATED NO. OF VISITS FOR SYMPTOMS (E) (16)[a]	DISCREPANCY BETWEEN ACTUAL AND ESTIMATED NO. OF VISITS (A−E)	SYMPTOMS-RESPONSE RATIO $\frac{(A-E)\,(100)^{b}}{E}$
Age (1)				
1-5	3,412	2,565	847	33**
6-17	7,529	6,728	801	12**
18-34	10,835	10,722	113	1
35-54	11,194	12,515	-1,321	-11**
55-64	7,289	7,854	-565	-7*
65 and over	9,811	10,163	-352	-3
Sex (2)				
Male	19,836	20,553	-717	-3*
Female	30,232	29,992	240	1
Race (3)				
White	44,672	44,507	165	0
Nonwhite	5,397	6,039	-642	-11*
Residence (4)				
SMSA, central city	15,813	15,569	244	2
SMSA, other urban	12,500	12,874	-374	-3
Urban, non-SMSA	6,470	6,301	169	3
Rural nonfarm	12,276	11,997	279	2
Rural farm	3,012	3,807	-795	-21**
Poverty level (5)				
Above	36,664	36,087	577	2
Below	13,404	14,459	-1,055	-7**
Regular source of care (6)				
None	1,756	3,966	-2,210	-56**
Clinic	8,782	9,049	-267	-3
GP	21,333	21,995	-662	-3
Specialist	15,395	13,051	2,343	18**
Total	50,070	50,547	-477	0

*Significant (P ≤ .05).
**Significant (P ≤ .001).
[a]These are the weighted number of visits for the sample and, thus, represent the *proportionate* distribution of visits among these subgroups in the population.
[b]See Chapter 3 for further discussion of computation of ratio and how test of significance was done on the index. In essence, a statistically significant finding means that the difference between the actual and estimated number of visits for symptoms by people in that population subgroup was greater than one would expect by chance, with a given probability of being in error (P ≤ .05 or P ≤ .001).

the medical necessity of the disability days, for which they want to take time off from work.

The differences between males and females with respect to whether they respond to symptoms as they should is not large. Men appear less apt to see a doctor when they need to than are women — though, as with the use-disability ratio, the differences between the sexes with respect to using services when the need arises is not as great, as when their respective need for care is not taken into account (as in Table 9).

Nonwhites see a doctor less often than they should, given the medical significance of their symptoms. Whites, on the other hand, appear to see a doctor as often as they need to, relative to the medically-evaluated severity of their complaints.

The people who live on farms in rural areas are much less likely to see a doctor when symptoms of illness arise than are people who live in cities or in rural areas, but not on farms.

Similarly, people below the poverty level see a doctor less often for symptoms than they should — while the nonpoor appear to see a doctor as often as is appropriate, given the medically-evaluated severity of their expressed complaints.

People who have no doctor as a regular source of care have substantially fewer visits to a doctor than they need, given the severity of the symptoms they report. People who have specialists, on the other hand, report more visits than the medical care experts deem necessary, considering the severity of their reported symptoms.

The findings on the symptoms-response ratio for the various race, residence, income and regular source of care subgroups affirm the differentials in access that were found in the analyses of the use-disability ratio and the other process and outcome indicators of access reported earlier. Nonwhites, rural farm people, the poor and those people who do not have a regular place they can go for medical advice or treatment, have less access to medical care than they "should," given the medically evaluated severity of their reported symptoms.

Table 17 points up the relative importance of some of these variables (regular source of care, race, poverty level) in influencing who gets care when they need it. People who report some regular source of care (clinic, GP or specialist) are more apt to use "appropriately" than those who have no place they generally go for medical advice or treatment. Among those who have a regular source of care, however, whites are much more likely than nonwhites to see a doctor for symptoms when they should. On the other hand, considering the people who have no usual place to go, nonwhites are somewhat more likely than the whites with no regular source of care to see a doctor as they should. And, in

TABLE 17
Symptoms-response ratio by regular source of care by race by poverty level

CHARACTERISTIC[a]	SYMPTOMS-RESPONSE RATIO
Regular source of care, white, above poverty level	6
white, below poverty level	2
nonwhite, below poverty level	− 6
nonwhite, above poverty level	−10
No regular source of care, nonwhite, below poverty level	−37
nonwhite, above poverty level	−41
white, above poverty level	−56
white, below poverty level	−64

[a]"Regular source of care" includes people who report either a clinic or medical doctor (GP or specialist) as their regular souce of medical care. "No regular source of care" means that they indicated *no* place that they went on a routine basis "for medical advice or treatment."

contrast to the whites, the poorer nonwhites are more apt than the nonpoor, nonwhites to see a doctor for symptoms.

These findings affirm that people who have no regular source of care are much less likely to see a doctor as they "should," when symptoms of illness occur. Among those who have no regular source of care, however, it appears that the nonwhite poor fare somewhat better than whites, with respect to getting care as they should when symptoms occur. All of those who have no usual place they go for care — whites or nonwhites, poor or nonpoor — see a doctor much less often than they "need to," however, given the medically-evaluated severity of the symptoms they experience.

Medical Severity Index

The implication in the discussion of the conventional use measures (Tables 9 and 10) and in the need-based use measures just examined is that, though some population subgroups delay longer than others in seeing a doctor, their need for care may actually be greater — so that when they do contact a physician, they may visit him more often.

The medical severity index permits this thesis to be tested more directly. The index is derived from physician evaluations of the medical urgency of the conditions that people who saw a physician in 1970 reported.

VARIABLE DESCRIPTION

The diagnoses reported by respondents were categorized with respect to whether they were for (1) preventive care, relief of symptoms or would not be affected by treatment, or whether (2) the person should or must see a doctor for such a condition. The first type of care was termed "elective" and the second "mandatory." Each respondent was classified according to whether all the diagnoses he reported were elective ("elective care only") or all were mandatory ("mandatory care only"), or if some of the conditions were of one kind and some the other ("elective and mandatory care").[5]

FINDINGS

For the sample as a whole, approximately one-third of the respondents fell into each of the three medical severity categories (see Table 18). A slightly larger percentage (37%) reported "elective types of care only."

In most cases, the population subgroups that were found to have the highest mean physician visits — among those who had at least one visit to a physician in 1970 (Table 10) — were also found to have the highest percent of people whose presenting conditions were "all mandatory."

Older adults 55-64 and the elderly, women, nonwhites, rural farm people, the poor and those who report clinics as their usual source of medical care had higher proportions of people whose diagnoses were mandatory than the other respective age, sex, race, etc. categories.[6]

Table 19 shows that, controlling for race and place of residence, the relationship of income to the distribution of responses on the medical severity index persists. The nonpoor have the highest rates of elective use and the poor the highest rates of mandatory use. The poor may average more visits to a doctor, once in the system, than the nonpoor (Table 10), but according to the medical severity index, the care they receive is also more apt to be medically urgent.

On the other hand, those groups that had the highest proportions seeking elective (non-mandatory) (Table 18) care were children under 18, males, people who live in SMSA's outside the central city, the nonpoor and people who have no regular source of care.

The finding that people who have no regular source of care are most apt to see a doctor for elective care only seems peculiar in the light of the findings on the use-disability and symptoms-response ratios — which suggest high levels of unmet need in this group. These latter measures include people who had need, but did not get into the system, however. People with no regular source of care, as a group, may be healthier, so

---

[5]See Chapter 3 for further discussion of how the medical severity index was constructed.

[6]With the exception of the residence and regular source of care categories, these were the same groups who had more visits to see a physician once they were in the system than their counterparts (See Table 10).

TABLE 18
Medical severity index by selected characteristics of population-at-risk

| CHARACTERISTIC | MEDICAL SEVERITY INDEX (17)[a] | | | |
	Percent elective care only	Percent elective and mandatory care	Percent mandatory care only	TOTAL PERCENT
Age (1)				
1-5	52	31	18	101[b]
6-17	54	23	23	100
18-34	34	34	32	100
35-54	33	35	31	99[b]
55-64	21	33	47	101[b]
65 and over	15	34	50	99[b]
Sex (2)				
Male	40	30	30	100
Female	35	33	33	101[b]
Race (3)				
White	37	33	31	101[b]
Nonwhite	39	23	38	100
Residence (4)				
SMSA, central city	35	32	33	100
SMSA, other urban	40	33	27	100
Urban, non-SMSA	37	31	32	100
Rural nonfarm	37	31	32	100
Rural farm	33	29	38	100
Poverty level (5)				
Above	38	32	30	100
Below	33	28	39	100
Regular source of care (6)				
None	46	24	31	101[b]
Clinic	33	31	36	100
GP	38	33	29	100
Specialist	37	32	32	101[b]
Total	37	32	31	100[c]

[a]See Chapter 3 for further discussion of how medical severity index was constructed.

[b]Does not add up to 100 (percent) because of rounding error.

[c]Percent table N is of U.S. population equals 65; percent who did not have a condition for which they saw the doctor in 1970 equals 35 (based on best estimate data).

that it is less central for them to establish a relationship with a regular doctor. When they do see the physician, however, more of them are apt to have less serious kinds of presenting complaints.

The medical severity index, then, serves to round out the picture of whether the people most in need of care get it or not. The conventional use measures suggested that some groups were less likely to contact a doctor than others, but once they did, they required more visits to get their medical problem resolved than those who had seen a doctor all along. The findings on the use-disability and symptoms-response indices showed that the poor, nonwhites and people on farms, for example, used fewer services than they "should," relative to their need for care. And the medical severity index further affirms that when these people do see a doctor though, it is much more apt to be for more medically severe kinds of presenting complaints.

People who had no regular source of care were much less apt to have contacted a doctor in 1970 (Table 9). This group also had lower rates of use relative to the disability days they experienced (Table 12) and they saw a doctor less often than they "should" in response to symptoms (Tables 15 and 16), then people who reported having some regular source of care. Further, according to the medical severity index, the people with no regular source of care who do see the doctor are most apt to have elective (non-mandatory) presenting complaints. One may conclude from these findings on the regular source of care variable, then,

TABLE 19
Medical severity index by poverty level by residence by race

		MEDICAL SEVERITY INDEX (17)					
		Percent with elective care only		Percent with elective and mandatory care		Percent with mandatory care only	
		POVERTY LEVEL (5)					
RACE (3)	RESIDENCE (4)	above	below	above	below	above	below
White	Urban	38	34	34	31	28	36
	Rural	37	31	32	27	31	42
Non-white	Urban	45	34	22	25	33	41
	Rural	34	33	25	23	41	44
Total		38	33	32	28	30	39

that healthier people may have no need for a regular source of care. The less healthy, who have no doctor they usually see, however, are apt to have high levels of unmet need.

CONTINUITY OF CARE

An important aspect of the utilization of health services is the continuity of care experienced by consumers. Richardson (1971), Solon, et al. (1967, 1969) and others, for example, introduce an episode of illness approach for examining the pattern and flow of patients through the health care system in response to illness. Gibson, et al. (1970), Satin and Duhl (1972), Weinerman, et al. (1966) and others point out that hospital emergency rooms are increasingly being used as primary medical care providers, because of the unavailability of physicians when the need arises. The pattern of response to episodes of illness and the tendency to use hospital emergency rooms for non-urgent conditions both serve as indicators of the degree of fragmentation and coordination of medical services.

In this section, several empirical indicators of these aspects of careseeking will be introduced and their relevance for evaluating the continuity of care discussed.

Use-Continuity Measures

VARIABLE DESCRIPTION

Several indices that describe the patterns of careseeking in response to a given episode of illness are: (1) the number of different providers seen to get the illness episode resolved; (2) the number of visits to each provider; and (3) the reason or source of referral to each provider.

FINDINGS

Shortell (1973) provides some preliminary data on these different indices for a subsample of the 1970 CHAS survey of women who had a pregnancy in 1970 (See Chapter 3 for description of questions used to elicit this information).

He found that the number of different sources seen for the pregnancy was highest for nonwhites, people in the inner city, and medium- and low-income groups and those who reported clinics as their usual source of care.

On the other hand, those groups that had the most mean visits per source were whites, people living in SMSA's outside the inner city, high-income groups and those who had specialists as their regular source of care.

Further, he found that the total number of sources was higher and visits per source lower for those who simply picked (or had their family pick) their most amount source of care, than those who were referred by their (or another) physician.

The use-continuity measures introduced here imply that (1) the more sources one has to see to get their medical problem resolved, (2) the fewer visits that occur to each source, and (3) the less formalized the process of referral to those sources, the less continuity of care he has.

These relationships are perhaps best considered in the context of episodes of serious illness, in which the precise steps taken by the patient to get his condition resolved, can be traced. In general, however, Shortell's findings for the pregnancy subsample from the 1970 study suggest that those groups that were found to have less access, in terms of some of the process and outcome indices examined earlier — nonwhites, inner-city people, the poor and those who have clinics as their usual source of care — also have the least continuity, when the number of sources, mean visits per source and means of referral to these sources are considered.

Use of Emergency Rooms for Primary Care

VARIABLE DESCRIPTION

The head of household and spouse of head in the 1970 CHAS survey were asked, for a list of selected medical conditions, what steps they would take to get the condition treated — call an ambulance, go to the hospital emergency room, see their doctor within three days, see their doctor within the month or do nothing.

The same panel of physicians, who were asked to evaluate the medical severity of the symptoms incorporated into the symptoms-response ratio (See Chapter 3), were also asked to indicate what the medically appropriate response to the five medical conditions should be.

For two of the conditions — sore throat with fever and a third headache in as many days — the physicians indicated that the person should see their doctor within three days. For the remaining three conditions, they suggested the person go to the hospital emergency room for treatment (See Chapter 3 for more detailed description of how these physician evaluations were determined).

The two conditions, for which the physicians thought people should see their doctor in a few days instead of going to a hospital emergency room, may be considered examples of care best rendered by primary care providers (frontline medical generalists or family practitioners).

In the analyses that follow, the percent who said they would go to emergency rooms to have these conditions treated will be compared with the percentages who said they would respond in some other way — see their doctor in three days (which the panel of physicians thought most appropriate), do nothing, etc., for different groups. In this way, those people that are most apt to go to emergency rooms to have their primary medical care needs met (and who, therefore, are apt to have less continuous and more fragmented medical care) can be identified.

FINDINGS

The majority of respondents chose that response which the panel of medical experts deemed most appropriate for the two conditions — seeing their doctor within three days (See Table 20).

In practically all categories of the population-at-risk, and for both medical conditions, people who had no regular doctor they saw for care were more apt to say they would go to a hospital emergency room for treatment than those who identified a particular doctor they usually saw for care. The percentages that said they would, as the panel of physicians thought appropriate, see a doctor in three days was consistently higher for people who had a particular physician they identified as their usual source of care. Further, the percent who said they would do nothing in response to these conditions was, for all age, sex, race, etc. categories, higher for those who could identify no particular doctor they routinely consulted for medical advice and treatment.

The impact of not having a usual source of care on whether or not a person would go to an emergency room for treatment, seems greatest for those population subgroups that, based on previous findings on the process and other outcome indicators, have the lowest levels of access to the system: nonwhites, rural dwellers, and people below the poverty level.

What these findings suggest, then, is that people who have no regular doctor they identify as their usual source of care are the most apt to go to hospital emergency rooms for conditions that may be best treated in a physician's office. And, as documented in the literature on the use of hospital emergency rooms as primary care centers (Kahn, et al., 1973; Satin, 1973), it is the nonwhites and the poor who are most likely to have this fragmented and poorly-coordinated kind of medical care.

CONSUMER SATISFACTION

As mentioned in the theoretical discussion of the access concept, consumers' subjective impressions of the medical care they receive is also important in evaluating their "access" to the health care delivery system.

Andersen, et al. (1971) point out that there are six primary dimensions of consumer satisfaction with care that might be evaluated: convenience, coordination, courtesy, information, out-of-pocket costs and qual-

TABLE 20
Percent using hospital emergency room for primary care by selected characteristics of population-at-risk by regular source of care

USE OF EMERGENCY ROOM FOR PRIMARY CARE (19)[a]

CHARACTERISTIC	REGULAR SOURCE OF CARE (6)[b]	Sore throat with fever					Third headache in three days				
		Call ambulance	Go to ER	See MD/ 3 days*	See MD/ month	Do nothing	Call ambulance	Go to ER	See MD/ 3 days*	See MD/ month	Do nothing
Age (1)											
Under 65	No regular doctor	1	18	52	1	28	1	14	57	8	21
	Regular doctor	0	11	68	1	20	0	8	70	5	17
65 and over	No regular doctor	1	15	48	1	35	1	8	57	3	31
	Regular doctor	0	10	68	1	21	0	8	73	3	15
Sex (2)											
Male	No regular doctor	1	18	52	1	29	1	13	56	7	23
	Regular doctor	1	12	65	1	21	1	10	67	5	18
Female	No regular doctor	1	18	52	1	29	1	13	57	7	22
	Regular doctor	0	10	69	1	19	0	7	72	5	16
Race (3)											
White	No regular doctor	1	14	54	0	31	0	11	59	7	23
	Regular doctor	0	10	68	1	21	0	7	71	5	17
Non-white	No regular doctor	2	40	38	2	17	2	26	42	10	21
	Regular doctor	1	22	66	2	10	1	15	67	5	12
Residence (4)											
Urban	No regular doctor	1	17	49	1	33	1	10	64	6	19
	Regular doctor	1	13	63	1	22	0	8	68	5	19
Rural	No regular doctor	1	18	53	1	27	1	14	54	8	24
	Regular doctor	0	10	70	1	19	0	8	72	5	16
Poverty level (5)											
Above	No regular doctor	1	15	5	0	29	0	10	62	9	20
	Regular doctor	0	10	69	1	20	0	7	71	5	17
Below	No regular doctor	2	24	43	2	29	2	11	44	4	29
	Regular doctor	1	15	63	1	20	0	8	68	5	17
Total[c]		1	12	65	1	22	0	9	68	5	18

*Indicates doctors' estimate of "medically appropriate response."

[a] The numbers in the columns represent the percent who say they would take each of the respective steps for that symptom. The percentages are computed so that in any row, the sum across a particular condition equals 100, subject to rounding error.

[b] The people with "no regular doctor" includes those who indicated they had no regular source of care or people who used clinics, but had no physician in particular they saw there. This permits all those who had no regular doctor they saw, to be considered together.

[c] Percent table N is of U.S. population equals 44: percent who had no regular doctor equals 55: NA equals 1.

ity. In the analyses that follow, responses representative of a family's satisfaction with these various aspects of their members' recent medical care encounters will be examined.

Special attention will be given to seeing if the respondent's own experience with the system, in term of some of the process indicators of access examined earlier — regular source of care, travel time, appointment waiting time, office waiting time, etc. — influence their subsequent levels of satisfaction or dissatisfaction with the system, i.e., are the people who have the least access, using these indices also the least satisfied?[7]

First, descriptive distributions of the percent dissatisfied with each aspect of care-seeking will be summarized. Then, Likert-type summated ratings scales of the dimensions that underlie these different attitudes will be introduced.

Percent Dissatisfied with Medical Care

VARIABLE DESCRIPTION

The 1970 CHAS survey included a health opinions questionnaire administered to the family head and spouse of each family. The total sample for the health opinion questionnaire included 4,966 people (unweighted). It was made up of:

Male head with spouse in household 37%
Male head without spouse in household 6%
Female head without spouse in household 16%
Wife of head 41%

Included on the questionnaire were a number of questions concerning satisfaction with health services, based on "the medical care you and those close to you have received over the past few years from doctors and hospitals."

Alpert, et al. (1967a:713) assert that, "On the basis of illness and health-related behavior, the family may be regarded as a meaningful unit which shows specific characteristics in maintaining health and in preventing, experiencing, and treating illness." More specifically, several studies cite the prevailing norm that the mother of a family has primary responsibility for assuming nursing care for the children and assessing their medical needs (Alpert, et al., 1967b; Wingert, et al., 1968). Hence,

---

[7]Notice that there is some transposition in the level of analyses — families and individuals — implied here. The satisfaction questions were asked of household heads and spouses of heads with respect to their *family's* recent contacts with doctors and hospitals. In the analyses that follow, then, we will deal with these respondents as *representatives* of their family's care-seeking experience, but also as *individuals* whose attitudes are apt to be influenced by the nature of their own recent medical care encounters.

in the analyses reported here, the respondents to the health opinions questionnaire whose attitudes are most apt to influence the family's medical care-seeking — wife of head, female head without spouse and male head without spouse — only, were included.[8] Further, only the people who themselves saw a doctor or were hospitalized in the year, or who came from families in which some member saw the doctor or was hospitalized, were chosen from the subset.[9] The findings reported here, then, reflect the responses of those family members most apt to be responsible for the family's health care and whose attitudes are most apt to be rooted in recent encounters with the health care system. The percent unsatisfied and very dissatisfied comprise the percent dissatisfied reported for each of the satisfaction items.

FINDINGS

In general, people were most dissatisfied with aspects of the convenience (availability of care after hours, office waiting time) and cost of medical care (See Table 21). The least dissatisfaction was expressed with respect to the courtesy shown them by providers and the overall quality of the medical care they received. These findings agree with those reported by Hulka, et al. (1971) in a study of a low-income population in North Carolina in 1969. The attitudes of respondents in that sample were, similarly, more favorable toward the personal and professional qualities of medical care providers and less favorable with respect to the cost and inconvenience of medical care.

The elderly reported lower levels of dissatisfaction with practically all aspects of the care-seeking process than the younger age groups.

Nonwhites, who are most apt to have the longest waiting times to get an appointment to see the doctor, were more dissatisfied than the whites, with the inconvenience and high costs of care. Whites were somewhat more dissatisfied than nonwhites with the doctor's concern for their overall health. Whites and nonwhites were equally pleased with the courtesy shown them by providers. Nonwhites were slightly more

---

[8]Using such a procedure, women are disproportionately represented in the analysis, i.e., approximately 92% of the responses are from women.

[9]Selecting on the basis of whether or not a person in the family had a visit to a doctor or a hospitalization in the year does not greatly reduce the number of people included in the sample. Twenty-five percent (25%) of the U.S. population are included, when only those who had some contact with the system are considered. Twenty-seven percent (27%) are involved when there is no selection on the basis of use. The findings for the subsample of families who saw a doctor or were hospitalized did not differ significantly from the results in which all families — regardless of whether there was a contact with the system — were considered. To separate out those who had the most intensive interaction with the system, maybe only families in which someone was hospitalized should be considered. Perhaps larger differences would emerge for this subsample, compared to those who had less intense or no contact(s) with the system.

TABLE 21
Percent dissatisfied with medical care by selected characteristics of population-at-risk

PERCENT DISSATISFIED WITH MEDICAL CARE (20)[a]

CHARACTERISTIC	Convenience — Office waiting time (b)	Convenience — Availability of care after hours (c)	Cost — Ease of getting to care (d)	Cost — Out-of-pocket cost (e)	Coordination — Getting all needs met at one place (l)	Coordination — Concern of doctors for overall health (k)	Coordination — Follow-up-care (j)	Courtesy — That shown by doctors (h)	Courtesy — That shown by nurses (i)	Medical Information — Information to choose doctor (m)	Medical Information — Information about what was wrong (f)	Medical Information — Information about treatment (g)	Overall Quality — Overall quality of care (a)
Age (1)													
Under 18[b]	*	*	*	*	*	*	*	*	*	*	*	*	*
18-34	38	40	12	40	21	18	7	10	10	21	18	9	8
35-54	34	41	10	37	22	15	6	6	9	16	13	7	9
55-64	34	47	13	36	16	16	5	6	4	7	13	8	8
65 and over	25	34	15	28	11	6	4	2	3	8	9	6	4
Sex (2)[c,d]													
Male	30	37	6	34	15	12	3	7	6	14	18	9	11
Female	34	41	12	37	19	16	6	7	7	16	14	8	8
Race (3)													
White	33	40	11	36	19	16	6	7	7	16	13	7	8
Nonwhite	45	51	23	46	18	10	9	7	7	14	20	14	13
Residence (4)													
SMSA, central city	35	42	15	35	19	14	5	8	8	18	16	10	8
SMSA, other urban	34	39	9	35	22	18	7	6	8	18	12	8	10
Urban, non-SMSA	29	35	9	39	19	14	7	4	7	12	11	7	7
Rural nonfarm	34	44	12	39	17	16	5	7	6	12	15	6	7
Rural farm	41	45	16	40	16	12	7	7	8	10	16	9	6
Poverty level (5)													
Above	32	41	10	35	20	16	6	7	7	16	14	7	8
Below	40	40	20	43	16	13	6	7	9	12	16	10	9
Total[d]	34	41	12	37	19	15	6	7	7	15	14	8	8

[a]The "percent dissatisfied" includes those who were "unsatisfied" or "very dissatisfied" with the respective aspects of care-seeking. The letter in parentheses after each item refers to its question number (see Chapter 3 for exact wording).

[b]The number of people under 18 years of age is less than 25 (unweighted).

[c]This and subsequent tables on satisfaction include only female heads of households, wife of male heads and male heads with no spouses of families in which one or more family members saw a doctor or were hospitalized during the preceding year. One family is represented by each respondent. Percent table N is of U.S. population equals 25: percent male heads of household, heads or spouses of families that had no visits to physician or hospital in 1970; family members who were not heads of household or spouses equal 74; N A equals 1.

[d]These results by sex are not very meaningful, given the disproportionate representation of women in this particular subsample.

dissatisfied than whites, however, with the information given about what was wrong, how it might be treated and the quality of the care they received.

Rural farm and SMSA, central city people, who had the least access — based on the process indices reported earlier — expressed the highest levels of dissatisfaction with the convenience of care. People in rural areas were least satisfied with costs. There was somewhat of a tendency for people in SMSA's outside the inner city (who are most apt to have specialists as their regular source of care) to express dissatisfaction with the ability to get one's needs met at one location and with the concern manifested by doctors for their overall health. People from SMSA's — both inside and outside the inner city — were equally dissatisfied with the information they had available to them for choosing a doctor. And inner-city and farm people were equally dissatisfied with the information provided by doctors about what was wrong with them and how it should be treated.

People whose income was below the poverty level were more likely than the nonpoor to be dissatisfied with the time they spent waiting to see a doctor, the ease of getting to his office and the out-of-pocket costs of care. The poor were found, in the analyses of the process indices reported earlier, to have the longest travel times to care and the longest waits to see a doctor. Their attitudes with respect to the convenience of care seem to reflect the discomfort they experienced. The nonpoor (like people in the "SMSA, other urban" category) had higher levels of dissatisfaction with the ability to get their needs met at one location and with the concern expressed by doctors for their overall health. This group may also have more referrals to specialists from their family doctors to get their problems resolved. However, there was apparently little difference between the poor and nonpoor with respect to satisfaction with the overall quality of medical care.

The preceding analyses have suggested that those groups which had the least access, based on the findings from the process indices reported earlier, were also least satisfied with the care-seeking process. The findings reported in Table 22 provide a more direct test of the impact of these factors on the consumers' satisfaction with the system.

People who had the least access, in terms of not having a particular physician that they saw for medical advice or treatment,[10] were least satisfied with the convenience and cost of medical services. Those persons with no regular source of care or specialists as their usual source of care were most dissatisfied with the ability to get their needs met at one location.

---

[10]This includes people who had no regular source of care and the clinic users who had no particular doctor they saw when they went for medical advice and treatment.

TABLE 22
Percent dissatisfied with medical care by process indices

PERCENT DISSATISFIED WITH MEDICAL CARE (20)[a]

PROCESS INDEX	Convenience			Cost	Coordination			Courtesy		Medical Information			Overall Quality
	Office waiting time (b)	Availability of care after hours (c)	Ease of getting to care (d)	Out-of-pocket cost (e)	Getting all needs met at one place (l)	Concern of doctors for overall health (k)	Follow-up care (j)	That shown by doctors (h)	That shown by nurses (i)	Information to choose doctor (m)	Information about what was wrong (f)	Information about treatment (g)	Overall quality of care (a)
Regular source of care (6)[b]													
None	41	48	17	43	31	20	6	16	12	26	23	12	14
Clinic-no MD name	50	41	17	40	20	25	12	18	15	22	26	11	16
Clinic-MD name	37	41	10	29	13	17	7	9	5	11	19	9	10
GP	32	40	12	35	17	13	6	6	8	13	14	8	7
Specialist	30	40	9	41	23	15	4	3	4	17	8	6	5
Travel time (7)													
Less than 15 minutes	31	37	5	33	18	14	7	6	7	15	12	8	7
15-30 minutes	36	43	15	38	18	17	5	6	8	14	15	8	7
31-60 minutes	38	44	30	46	18	11	5	5	5	15	12	7	7
More than one hour	39	43	31	35	13	18	8	8	5	20	20	9	14
Appointment or walk-in visit (8)													
Appointment	31	39	11	35	20	15	6	6	6	15	13	8	7
Walk-in	40	43	12	40	14	14	7	7	10	12	15	8	10
Appointment waiting time (9)													
Same day to 2 days	27	35	11	35	19	13	6	4	6	14	11	8	7
3 days to 2 weeks	35	43	11	36	16	17	4	6	6	13	14	4	7
More than 2 weeks	47	52	15	39	34	22	11	17	7	27	18	13	7
Office waiting time (10)													
Immediate	15	25	6	19	13	11	6	4	6	11	7	2	5
1 to 30 minutes	20	35	10	33	18	12	5	5	6	13	11	7	5
31 to 60 minutes	38	41	10	40	17	19	7	6	7	16	16	8	10
More than one hour	70	57	20	47	21	19	6	10	10	18	18	10	13
Total[c]	34	41	12	37	19	15	6	7	7	15	14	8	8

[a] The "percent dissatisfied" includes those who were "unsatisfied" or "very dissatisfied" with the respective aspect of care-seeking. The letter in parentheses after each item refers to its question number (see Chapter 3 for exact wording).

[b] The "clinic-no MD name" category refers to people who reported a clinic as their usual source of care, but did not have a particular doctor they usually saw at the clinic. The "clinic-MD name" people reported having a doctor they usually saw.

[c] See footnote c (Table 21) for description of who is included in this table. In addition, those who reported "other" or no answer for the regular source of care variable are excluded. Only those who had a regular source are included in the findings for the other process indices — travel time, etc.

People who went to clinics, but had no doctor they usually saw, were least satisfied with doctors' concern for their overall health, the follow-up care they received, and the courtesy shown them by doctors and nurses. The people who had no medical practitioner they identified as their own were more dissatisfied than those with a family doctor, with respect to the information available to them for choosing a physician, the information about their ailment and the proper treatment for it, and the overall quality of the care they received.

Further, the people most dissatisfied with the convenience of care were those who had to travel more than 15 minutes to reach their regular source of care. There was a tendency for people who had the least access — in terms of having to travel more than an hour to reach their usual source of care — to be most dissatisfied with aspects of coordination, physician courtesy, the information provided them about how to choose doctors and the condition they had, and the overall quality of care they received.

The people who just walked in to see the doctor and those with appointments who had to wait more than a week to be scheduled were generally the most dissatisfied with all aspects of care-seeking — convenience, cost, coordination, etc.

A similar pattern may be seen in terms of office waiting time. People who had the "least access," i.e., had to wait more than an hour to see the doctor, were most dissatisfied with all dimensions of the process of receiving care.

Summated Ratings Scales of Satisfaction

The preceding analyses have provided some insights into the dimensions of medical care-seeking with which consumers are most dissatisfied and the influence of their actual contacts with the system on satisfaction. To provide a more integrated measure of these dimensions and the degree to which people are dissatisfied, the items just reviewed will be collapsed into Likert-type summary scales,[11] in the analyses that follow.

VARIABLE DESCRIPTION

The findings on the percent dissatisfied with medical care just reported suggest that people in general are least satisfied with the cost and convenience of medical care and more satisfied with those aspects that pertain more directly to the characteristics and behavior of the providers — coordination, courtesy, medical information, overall quality. Hulka,

---

[11]See A.L. Edwards, *Techniques of Attitude Scale Construction*, New York: Appleton-Century-Crofts, Inc., 1957, for a discussion of the Likert method of summated ratings, pp. 149-171.

et al. (1971), as mentioned previously, found similar results on their Thurstone scales of consumer satisfaction with cost-convenience, professional competence and personal qualities of providers.

In our theoretical discussion of the access concept, we noted two main aspects of the organization of the delivery system, that should be considered in describing access to the system — entry and structure. The differentials in the level of satisfaction with care found in these preliminary analyses seem to describe these same two aspects of the system. The cost and convenience dimensions of satisfaction more directly concern the process of gaining entry to the system, for example, while coordination, courtesy, medical information and quality of care refer more to the organization and behavior of the medical care providers themselves.

In the analyses that follow, therefore, two main satisfaction scales will be developed that integrate the relevant satisfaction items into dimensions of consumer attitudes toward (1) the process of entry to the system, and (2) the organization and behavior of the medical care providers themselves.

FINDINGS

The cost and convenience satisfaction items reflect attitudes toward the process of gaining entrance to the system (Table 23). The coordination, courtesy, medical information and quality of care items relate more to consumers' satisfaction with how the system itself is organized.

Table 23 shows the inter-correlations among these different satisfaction items. With the exception of the ease of getting to care item, the cost and convenience items are more highly correlated with one another than with the other items: coordination, courtesy, etc. Similarly, except for the question about getting all one's needs met at one place, the coordination, courtesy, and medical information items have higher correlations with one another than with the cost and convenience questions. These preliminary correlations, then, provide empirical support for, what seem to be central dimensions of satisfaction with care — "cost-convenience" and "provider-characteristic" type dimensions.

A factor analytic solution of this correlation matrix (iterated Alpha solution with squared multiple correlations as communality estimates), done by John Ware, Project Director, Measuring Health Concepts Research Testing Center, Southern Illinois University, also provides evidence for the existence of these two dimensions. The factor loadings of each satisfaction item for the two factors may be seen in Table 24.

This factor analytic solution similarly affirms that, with the exception of the ease of getting to care item, the other convenience and the cost item loads high on the same factor (Factor 1). And, except for the item

TABLE 23
Pearson correlation coefficients among satisfaction items

PEARSON CORRELATION COEFFICIENTS AMONG SATISFACTION ITEMS (20)

CHARACTERISTIC	Convenience			Cost	Coordination			Courtesy		Medical Information			Overall Quality
	Office waiting time (b)	Availability of care after hours (c)	Ease of getting to care (d)	Out-of-pocket cost (e)	Getting all needs met at one place (l)	Concern of doctors for overall health (k)	Follow-up care (j)	That shown by doctors (h)	That shown by nurses (i)	Information to choose doctor (m)	Information about what was wrong (f)	Information about treatment (g)	Overall quality of care (a)
Convenience													
Office waiting time (b)	1.00												.40
Availability or care after hours (c)	.45	1.00											.40
Ease of getting to care (d)	.28	.35	1.00										.34
Cost													
Out-of-pocket cost (e)	.39	.42	.31	1.00									.39
Coordination													
Getting all needs met at one place (l)	.31	.37	.32	.33	1.00								.35
Concern of doctors for overall health (k)	.35	.35	.31	.37	.53	1.00							.55
Follow-up care (j)	.27	.31	.35	.29	.39	.58	1.00						.50
Courtesy													
Courtesy shown by doctors (h)	.34	.32	.35	.32	.40	.61	.58	1.00					.57
Courtesy shown by nurses (i)	.34	.30	.31	.30	.37	.49	.54	.64	1.00				.41
Medical information													
Information to choose doctor (m)	.33	.38	.32	.30	.49	.49	.44	.44	.42	1.00			.44
Information about what was wrong (f)	.34	.38	.36	.35	.43	.57	.52	.58	.43	.52	1.00		.55
Information about treatment (g)	.30	.35	.35	.31	.40	.52	.53	.54	.44	.47	.67	1.00	.49
Overall quality													
Overall quality of care (a)													1.00

TABLE 24
Factor analysis of satisfaction items[a]

| | FACTORS | |
| | Factor 1 | Factor 2 |
	Factor Loadings	
Convenience		
Office waiting time (b)	.57159	.23304
Availability of care after hours (c)	.68723	.20993
Ease of getting to care (d)	.38800	.33485
Cost		
Out-of-pocket cost (e)	.56319	.23749
Coordination		
Getting all needs met at one place (l)	.39851	.45536
Concern of doctors for overall health (k)	.33096	.69267
Follow-up care (j)	.21536	.71432
Courtesy		
Courtesy shown by doctors (h)	.24124	.76432
Courtesy shown by nurses (i)	.26617	.60810
Medical Information		
Information to choose doctor (m)	.38050	.53187
Information about what was wrong (f)	.34337	.67845
Information about treatment (g)	.29015	.66088
Overall Quality		
Overall quality of care (a)	.42137	.55358

[a]This factor analytic solution was done on the correlation matrix in Table 23 by John Ware, Project Director, Measuring Health Concepts Research Training Center, Southern Illinois University. The solution was an iterated Alpha solution with squared multiple correlations as communality estimates. Ware cautioned, however, that additional analyses should be conducted to fully assess the dimensionality of the matrix, i.e., considerations of the distributions of reponses to the items, etc.

concerning getting all one's needs met at one place, the coordination, courtesy and medical information dimensions load highest on a second factor (Factor 2).

The average inter-item correlation (Table 23) for the cost-convenience items, excluding the "ease of getting to care" question is .39. For the items suggested for a "provider-characteristic" scale, the average inter-item correlation (excluding the "getting all needs met at one place" item) is .52. The average inter-item correlations for these two scales, considered separately, is higher than the average of the correlations of the items in the cost-convenience scale *with* the items in the provider-characteristic scale (.33). This finding, too, further suggests the utility of considering these "cost-convenience" and "provider-characteristic" item-clusters separately.

In general, the items that describe most directly the actual "laying on of hands" by the physician — the coordination, courtesy and medical information provided by the doctor — are most highly correlated with the consumer's attitudes toward the overall quality of care he received (Table 23). The factor analytic solution (Table 24), further, shows that the quality of care item loads higher on the provider-characteristic than the cost-convenience scale. Consumer evaluations of quality then, seem to be more highly related to the behavior and characteristics of the providers themselves, than to the cost and inconvenience experienced getting there.

To proceed with the construction of summary scales, using the Likert method of summated ratings, the response on the different items (range 1 to 4 — very satisfied to very dissatisfied) thought to reflect an underlying scale should be summed to obtain a total score for each individual. The values assigned to each of the response categories (1 to 4) for each item represent the level of satisfaction or dissatisfaction perceived by the respondent with respect to that aspect of care-seeking. The higher his summary score for a cluster of items, the more dissatisfied he is, then, with that dimension of obtaining care.

Before finalizing the items to be included in the different scales, however, an item analysis procedure is necessary to insure that every item included in the scale is related to the underlying attitudes represented by the scale. The inter-correlation analysis has provided some documentation of which items seem to meaningfully cluster into scales. To provide a more direct test of the internal consistency of the items included in the respective scales, however, the correlation of each item which is summed into the scale, with the total score for that scale (corrected for overlap) should be obtained. The higher the correlation coefficient between that item and the total score (excluding item itself from total) the more apt the item is to be related to the underlying attitude represented by that cluster of items.[12]

Table 25 shows the correlation of each of the items included in a cost-convenience and provider-characteristic scale with the total score on that scale for each individual (corrected for overlap). The two items found to have low inter-correlations with other items in their respective clusters (Table 23) — the ease of getting to care and the ability to get one's medical needs met at one place — also have the lowest correlations with the total scores on the respective scales. As these items are not as strongly related to the underlying attitudes reflected in the different scales, they will not be included in the final formulation of the scales.[13]

The scores for each individual on the final summary scales (See Table 26) are constructed by summing the values on all items included in the scale and dividing by the number of items.[14] The possible range of values for each scale, then, is between 1 and 4 with higher values indicating greater levels of dissatisfaction. Thus, a score of 4 would indicate that everyone in the group was "very dissatisfied" and a score of 1 would indicate that everyone was "very satisfied."

The most salient generalization to be made from the findings on the scales themselves is that, as suggested in the analysis of the percent dissatisfied with care, people *are less* pleased with the cost and convenience aspects of care-seeking, than with the personal and professional qualities of the medical care providers themselves. The time that one has to travel to care and whether or not he generally has an appointment to

---

[12]Another method to evaluate the internal consistency of the scale and the items included in it is to determine which of the items in a scale discriminate most clearly between the high and low scorers on the total scale. The responses of those subjects whose total scores are in the upper quarter and the responses of those in the lower quarter may be analyzed, using the difference-of-means t-test, for example, to determine for each item, whether the mean score on this statement is significantly different for the high-score and low-score groups. Items that do not show and those who score low on the total test are eliminated. Edwards (1957), however, argues that a correlation analysis, such as the one used here, is equally effective in determining which items should be retained in a Likert-type scale.

[13]The overall quality of care item is not included in either of the scales. The items described by the "provider-characteristic" dimension were found to be most highly correlated with satisfaction with the overall quality of care (See Table 23). No new information is added, in particular, by combining this item with others, however. Conceptually, the aspects of care described in the "provider-characteristic" dimension may be considered to be what the respondent *means* when he appraises the "overall quality" of care he received. The correlation between this variable and the scale (when the variable itself is not included in the scale) is .64. Its correlation with the cost-convenience dimension is .51.

[14]The total score was divided by the number of items, to produce values that had the same range (1-4) on each scale.

TABLE 25
Pearson correlation coefficients of satisfaction items in sumary scales with total scale scores

	SATISFACTION SUMMARY SCALES (20)	
	Cost-convenience	Provider-characteristic
SATISFACTION ITEMS (18)[a]	Pearson correlation coefficients	
Convenience		
Office waiting time (b)	.32	
Availability of care after hours (c)	.42	
Ease of getting to care (d)	.25[b]	
Cost		
Out-of-pocket cost (e)	.35	
Coordination		
Getting all needs met at one place (l)		.39[b]
Concern of doctors for overall health (k)		.52
Follow-up care (j)		.54
Courtesy		
Courtesy shown by doctors (h)		.48
Courtesy shown by nurses (i)		.44
Medical Information		
Information to choose doctor (m)		.49
Information about what was wrong (f)		.48
Information about treatment (g)		.49

[a]The items for which correlations appear are the ones included in the original "cost-convenience" and "provider-characteristic" scales, respectively.
[b]This item will be eliminated from the final scale.

TABLE 26
Scores on satisfaction summary scales by process indices by poverty level

	SATISFACTION SUMMARY SCALES (20)[a]			
	Cost-convenience		Provider-characteristic	
	POVERTY LEVEL (5)			
PROCESS INDEX	Above	Below	Above	Below
Regular source of care (6)				
None	2.5	2.5	2.0	2.0
Clinic-no MD name	2.4	2.6	2.0	2.1
Clinic-MD name	2.3	2.4	1.9	1.9
GP	2.3	2.3	1.9	1.8
Specialist	2.3	2.4	1.8	1.9
Travel time (7)				
Less than 15 minutes	2.3	2.3	1.9	1.9
15 to 30 minutes	2.4	2.4	1.9	1.9
31 to 60 minutes	2.4	2.4	1.9	1.9
More than one hour	2.3	2.3	1.9	2.0
Appointment or walk-in visit (8)				
Appointment	2.3	2.4	1.9	1.9
Walk-in	2.4	2.4	1.9	1.9
Appointment waiting time (9)				
Same day to 2 days	2.3	2.3	1.9	1.8
3 days to 2 weeks	2.3	2.5	1.9	1.9
More than 2 weeks	2.5	2.4	2.0	2.1
Office waiting time (10)				
Immediate	1.9	2.1	1.6	1.7
1 to 30 minutes	2.2	2.2	1.9	1.8
31 to 60 minutes	2.4	2.4	1.9	2.0
More than one hour	2.7	2.7	2.0	2.0
Total	2.4	2.4	1.9	1.9

[a]The items included in the final scales are as follows: cost-convenience — office waiting time, availability of care after hours, out-of-pocket cost; provider-characteristic — concern of doctors for overall health, follow-up care, courtesy shown by doctors, courtesy shown by nurses, information to choose doctor, information about what was wrong, information about treatment. The higher the score, the more dissatisfaction expressed. See text for description of how the scales were created.

see the doctor seem to have little effect on people's attitudes toward care. People who have no regular source of care or go to clinics, but have no doctor they usually see, do, however, seem to express somewhat more dissatisfaction with both the cost-convenience and the provider-characteristic dimensions, than those who have a particular doctor they usually see. There is a tendency for people who have to wait more than two weeks to get an appointment with their doctor to be more dissatisfied. People who have the longest waits to see a physician, once in his office, consistently express the highest level of dissatisfaction with both the cost and convenience of care and the characteristics and behavior of the providers themselves. This differential persists across income levels.

The striking similarity of satisfaction levels between the poor and the nonpoor when the process indices are used as controls should be noted. For both scales — cost-convenience and provider-characteristic — the majority of the scale scores for the poor and nonpoor are the same and in no case do they vary by more than .2. These findings suggest that the process indices do account for much of the difference in dissatisfaction among population groups noted in Table 21. For example, while the poor were more dissatisfied with waiting time and out-of-pocket costs in Table 21, we find in Table 26, no difference in cost-convenience satisfaction in three of the four groups when we control for waiting time. The ability of the process indices to account for differences in dissatisfaction among various population groups should be examined further.

In summary, this review of measures of consumers' satisfaction with medical care suggests that the majority of the American public are relatively satisfied with the medical care that they and their families receive. Those who are disenchanted are most displeased with the cost and inconvenience of medical care and less so with the characteristics and performance of the providers themselves. Summary scales of satisfaction, such as the ones developed here, permit more clear-cut generalizations regarding people's satisfaction with some overall dimensions of care-seeking. Certain groups who had the least access in terms of some of the process indices — especially those who had no regular doctor, had to wait more than two weeks to get an appointment or wait more than an hour to see a doctor, once in his office — were found to be least satisfied with both the cost-convenience and provider-characteristic aspects of medical care.

SUMMARY AND EVALUATION OF OUTCOME INDICES

We introduced the discussion of empirical indicators of the access concept with the description and presentation of data on selected process indicators of access to the medical care system that, in our theoretical model of the concept, were hypothesized to influence the utilization of health services by the population-at-risk and their subsequent satisfaction (or dissatisfaction) with the medical care they received. We found that certain groups in the population — nonwhites, rural farm and inner city residents, the poor and people who used clinics as their regular source of medical care, for example — were apt to have less access to the system, in terms of some of these process indicators — long travel times to care, walk-in visits rather than appointments, long waiting times to get an appointment, or to see the doctor, once in his office — than others.

In the section just concluded, we have, for these same population groups, described and presented findings on some key outcome-type indices of the access concept — empirical indicators of aspects of the utilization of health services and consumer satisfaction with care, that were introduced in the theoretical discussion of the access framework.

Four main kinds of indicators were reviewed: (1) conventional use measures; (2) need-based use measures; (3) continuity of care indices; and (4) satisfaction with care scales. The conventional use measures — percent (not) seeing a doctor and mean physician visits overall and for those with one or more visits — provide information on the contact and volume aspects of health services utilization. The need-based use measures — use-disability ratio, symptoms-response ratio and medical severity index[15] — integrate these contact and volume measures with people's actual need for care. Through such indices, an assessment of whether the people who really need care receive it or not, can be made. The continuity indices — use-continuity measures and the use of hospital emergency rooms for primary care needs — reflect the pattern and coordination of health care. And the satisfaction scales permit the subjective perceptions of consumers, with respect to the care they received, to be summarized.

Table 27 shows that many of the same groups who are found to have less access, in terms of some of the process indicators of the concept, were also found to have the least access, when the outcome-type measures of the concept were used.

Children 6-17 were least apt to see the doctor. When people's actual need for care was considered, however, it was the middle-aged and older adults who had the least access, i.e., the most unmet medical need. The

---

[15]Perhaps this measure is less appropriately considered as an index of access to care, than simply a descriptor of the "purpose" of care-seeking. It describes, for those who did see the doctor, whether their visits were most apt to be "mandatory" or "elective" in nature.

TABLE 27
Summary of population groups with "least access"[a] according to outcome indicators

CHARACTERISTIC	CONVENTIONAL USE MEASURES		NEED-BASED USE MEASURES			CONTINUITY OF CARE		CONSUMER SATISFACTION (20)	
	Percent not seeing MD (11)	Mean MD visits overall (12)	Use-disability ratio (13, 14)	Symptoms-response ratio (15, 16)	Medical severity[b] index (17)	Use-continuity measures (18)	Use of ER for primary care (19)	Cost-convenience	Provider characteristic
Age (1)	Children 6-17	Children 6-17	Adults 55-64	Adults 35-54	Adults 65 and over	c	Children and adults under 65	Children and adults under 65 [d]	Children and adults under 65 [d]
Sex (2)	Males	Males	No difference	Males	Females	c	Males		
Race (3)	Nonwhites	Nonwhites	Nonwhites	Nonwhites	Nonwhites	Nonwhites	Nonwhites	Nonwhites	No difference
Residence (4)	Rural farm	Rural farm	Rural farm	Rural farm	Rural farm	SMSA inner city	SMSA inner city and rural nonfarm	SMSA inner city and rural farm	No difference
Poverty level (5)	Below	No difference	Below	Below	Below	Below	Below	Below	
Regular source of care (6)	No regular source	No regular source	No regular source	No regular source	Clinic	Clinic	No regular source	No regular source	No regular source

[a]The groups with the "least access" are determined as follows for each index: (11) had highest proportion of people with *no* MD visit; (12) had fewest mean MD visits overall; (13, 14) had lowest score on use-disability ratio; (15, 16) had lowest score on symptoms-response ratio; (17) had highest proportion with "mandatory care only"; (18) had most sources of care, fewest visits per source, and informal, non-professional referral to most amount source; (19) had highest proportion of people using ER for non-urgent conditions; (20) had highest "percent dissatisfied" or highest values on satisfaction summary scales.

[b]Perhaps this measure is less appropriately considered as an index of access to care, than as a description of the "purpose" of care-seeking.

[c]Information on this variable was not applicable for particular subsample analyzed — pregnant women.

[d]Information on this variable was not applicable because of the disproportionate representation of women in the subsample analyzed.

elderly who saw the doctor were more apt than the other age groups to have serious (non-elective) kinds of presenting complaints. It was the people under 65, however, who were more likely to go to a hospital emergency room, if they needed primary medical attention. And it was the people under 65 who were least satisfied with all aspects of care-seeking, cost-convenience and the characteristics and performance of providers.

Males were apt to have lower rates of use overall than females. When the need for care was taken into account, however, the relationship of sex to these outcome indicators was less clear-cut. The differences by sex, using the use-disability and symptoms-response ratio were insignificant. Women were more apt than men to have more serious kinds of presenting complaints, when they did see the doctor, however. Men used the hospital emergency room for primary medical care more often than women.

Nonwhites consistently had fewer physician contacts and visits, less use relative to their actual need for care, more fragmented and ill-coordinated patterns of care and greater levels of dissatisfaction with the cost and convenience of services overall than whites.

As with the process indices, it was the rural farm and inner city residents who had the least access in terms of the outcome indicators of the concept. People who lived on farms in rural areas had the lowest rates of physician use and the lowest levels of use relative to their real need for care. People in inner cities were apt to have the most fragmented and ill-coordinated patterns of care. And it was the inner city and rural farm dwellers who were most dissatisfied with the cost and convenience of services in general.

People whose income was below the poverty level were less apt to contact a doctor than the nonpoor. The use of services overall was quite similar for the poor and the nonpoor, however. But when their actual need for care was taken into account, it was the poor who used fewer services, relative to their need, than the nonpoor. People whose income was below the poverty level had more fragmented and less continuous care than the nonpoor and were, also, much more dissatisfied, overall, with the out-of-pocket costs and inconvenience of medical services.

People who had no particular place they went for medical advice and treatment were apt to have the fewest visits to a physician and, according to the need-based access indices, have the highest levels of unmet medical need. People who routinely went to clinics for medical advice or treatment were apt to have the most serious presenting complaints when they did see a doctor. Clinic users and people with no regular physician were apt to have the most discontinuous care. And clinic users who had no particular physician that they saw or people who had no regular place they usually went for care, were most dissatisfied with all aspects of care-seeking — both its cost and convenience and the characteristics and performance of the providers themselves.

In the summary and evaluation of the process indicators of the access concept, each index was discussed with respect to its validity, reliability, variance, ease of collection, ease of computation, ease of interpretation and mutability. In this section, these same criteria will be applied to evaluate the outcome indicators of access just reviewed.

All of the outcome measures seem to fare well with respect to the validity of the differences they express. The conventional use measures have appeared frequently in the health services research literature and have yielded consistent and interpretable differences in access to health care over time.

The need-based use measures provide more direct estimates of unmet medical need in the population. With respect to the face validity criterion, the findings on the use-disability, symptoms-response and medical severity indices all make sense, in the light of what we know of the utilization experience and need of the respective population subgroups. These measures also seem valid, with respect to the content validity criterion. In focusing on whether the people who need care receive it or not, the need-based use measures serve to highlight an issue of central concern for evaluating access to the health care system — do the people most in need of care receive it or not? These indices do not, however, reflect the medical needs of diseases that are often asymptomatic and non-disabling in the early stages, such as malignant neoplasms, diabetes, hypertension, etc. Estimates of this source of need are very difficult to derive from household interview data though, and are best captured using direct physical examination of the population (Donabedian, 1973).

As mentioned in the theoretical discussion of the access concept, not only whether or not one sees a physician and how often he sees him are important in evaluating access to the system, but also the pattern and degree of coordination of the care he receives. The use-continuity measures and the index of the use of hospital emergency rooms for primary care both serve as meaningful descriptors of these aspects of care seeking — as they sample the universe of items generally deemed relevant to consider in evaluating the continuity of the medical care process.

The satisfaction scales were intended to yield summary measures of people's attitudes toward some general dimensions of medical care. The satisfaction measures developed appear to reflect differentials in consumer satisfaction that parallel discrepancies in access found for the other outcome and process indicators. The differences in satisfaction among the different population subgroups make sense, given what we know of the experiences of the respective groups with the health care delivery system. As Somers (1971) and others point out, these subjective or qualitative aspects of care-seeking are important in evaluating people's access to the health care system.

With respect to the reliability of these different outcome indices, the conventional use measures have been found to yield meaningful and consistent results over different times and situations.

Some material is provided on the inter-rater and intra-rater reliability of the physicians' estimates of severity for the symptoms-response index in Chapter 3. The use-disability and medical severity measures are new indexes, which, to fully test the reliability and stability of their findings, should be computed for the same subgroups in different populations.

The use-continuity measures are relatively new indexes, also. Work is presently being done to apply these same measures to a subsample of the 1970 CHAS survey, who experienced a major illness in the year, to see if they yield comparable findings. The findings from the literature on the use of the emergency room as a primary care center by certain groups was affirmed, using our index of respondents' hypothetical response to selected medical conditions.

The satisfaction scales reflect differences found in previous studies regarding consumer satisfaction with comparable dimensions of care-seeking (Andersen, et al., 1971; Hulka, et al., 1971).

As mentioned in the evaluation of the process indices, the "variance" of an estimate refers to its ability to detect "true differences over time and place." Based on the preliminary findings on both the well-tried conventional use measures and the new need-based, continuity and satisfaction indices, the outcome indices of access introduced here do appear to reflect meaningful variability among groups.

To be most meaningful to policy makers, the information required to construct the various indices should be fairly easy to collect.

The questions required to elicit information on the conventional use measures are relatively straightforward ones.

Perhaps the catchment period (two weeks) used to elicit information for construction of the use-disability ratio, should be extended, because of the small number of people who report disability days in that time interval. The trade-offs between extending the reporting period, to include more people, and providing a time interval, such that people can accurately recall their recent medical care experiences, should be weighed.

Collecting information from physicians for the symptoms-severity ratings and medical severity index requires some extra amount of time and resources. Perhaps norms should be collected from a large sample of physicians in different types of medical care settings, tested (much as was done with the 40 University of Chicago physicians' rankings) and refined, to provide a single set of standards that could be validly applied to a variety of populations or settings. New physician severity information should not have to be collected in every new situation in which the index is applied.

The continuity of care questions are perhaps best phrased in the context of an episode of illness — whom did the patient see first and why; what was the disposition of his case at that source; and how many other sources did he see to get the condition resolved and how many visits did he have to each source, etc. Providing such a context may enhance the patient's recall of his medical care encounters and permit a more full-blown description of the continuity of care he experienced with respect to that particular episode of care-seeking.

The satisfaction items in the 1970 CHAS survey were asked only of the head of household or wife of head — and in the context of the family's recent medical care encounters. Though there may be problems associated with asking such questions of the very young or very old members of the household, querying only the heads of the household or their spouses, with respect to the family's recent encounters yields rather diffuse information with respect to individuals' contacts with the system. More attention should, perhaps, be directed to designing items that are sensitive to the level of satisfaction or dissatisfaction experienced by particular individuals in specific, identifiable and recent contacts with the medical care system. The precise dimensions that gave rise to these satisfaction levels should be identified. In this way, policy makers can more meaningfully identify those aspects of the system that should be altered, to improve consumers' satisfaction with it.

Another attribute of a good access index is that it be fairly easy to compute. Relatively straightforward algorithms could be provided for the computation of each of the outcome measures introduced here. The most difficulty may be presented by those measures that attempt to integrate some external norm of appropriateness with respondents' actual behavior. As mentioned previously, some additional amount of effort is required to collect and determine these medically-derived criteria.

Any useful index of access should be capable of being rather straightforwardly interpreted. The conventional use measures reflect who used the most services and who the least. The need-based use measures show who used the most services and who the least, relative to their actual need for care. The continuity measures inform us about the pattern and coordination of care respondents received. And the satisfaction scales reflect who was pleased and who displeased — and with what aspects of medical care.

A final criteria that should be used to evaluate a meaningful index of access is the mutability of the phenomenon that it reflects. Each of the measures introduced here describe characteristics of the care-seeking process that may well be altered by the health care delivery system, or by the behavior or characteristics of the consumers, who participate in it, to improve their access to the system.

3

Methodological Notes

Introduction

This chapter provides a more extensive description of some of the methods used in collecting the data and computing the indexes reported in previous chapters. Definitions of the variables and the sample design used in this study are presented, as is background information on the construction of the symptoms-response ratio, medical severity index, and evaluation of the "appropriate" use of hospital emergency rooms.

Definitions of Variables

CHARACTERISTICS OF POPULATION-AT-RISK

Age (1)

Age is reported as of December 31, 1970. Children under one year of age are excluded from these analyses.

Sex (2)

There are no missing data on sex.

Race (3)

Each family member is coded according to the race of the main respondents. The census definitions of white and nonwhites are used. People of Mexican or Spanish descent are coded "white," — American Indians, Orientals and blacks as "nonwhite."

Residence (4)

The residence of each person in the sample is classified according to U.S. Census designation of the locality in which the residence is located plus the interviewer's description of the dwelling unit and locality:

(1) SMSA, central city — residence in the urban part of a Standard Metropolitan Statistical Area (SMSA) according to the Census, which is also designated by the interviewer as "inside the largest city in the primary unit";

(2) SMSA, other urban — same as (1) above except interviewer did not describe dwelling as "inside largest city";

(3) Urban, non-SMSA — residence in urban localities which are not part of an SMSA;

(4) Rural nonfarm — residence in areas defined as rural by the Census, which are not described as "farms" by the interviewer;

(5) Rural farm — residence in areas defined as rural by the Census, which are described as "farms" by the interviewer.

Poverty Level (5)

A family was considered to be "below" the poverty level if they reported their income to be less than the following amounts for a given family size:

Family Size	Monthly	Yearly	Weekly
1	$ 220	$ 2,600	$ 50
2	310	3,700	70
3	370	4,500	85
4	470	5,700	110
5	550	6,600	130
6	620	7,500	145
7+	760	9,100	175

These breakdowns were determined using Bureau of Labor Statistics cutting points.

Process Indices

Regular Source of Care (6)

The respondent's regular source of care is based on the response to the question, "Is there a particular medical person or clinic (PERSON) usually goes to when sick or for advice about health?" and follow-up question, "is that a clinic, a regular family doctor, some type of specialist, a chiropractor, or what?"

"None" means that there is no "particular" medical person or clinic the individual usually goes to when sick or for advice about health.

"Clinic" refers to the fact that the individual designates a "clinic" rather than an individual practitioner. Within the "clinic" category, further distinction is made according to an additional follow-up question, "Does (PERSON) go to a particular doctor at this clinic?", with responses signifying the following:

Yes — particular doctor's name given

No — no particular doctor indicated

The "GP" and "specialist" designations are based on how the physician classifies himself for the A.M.A. directory. All reported, specialties, including internal medicine, pediatrics and obstetrics-gynecology, are designated as "specialist" in our code. If the number was not found in the directory, the classification was based on whether the respondent said the person was their "regular family doctor" (GP) or "some type of specialist."

The "other" category (which is not reported in these analyses) includes those who cite an osteopath, chiropractor, podiatrist, visiting nurse, homeopath, naturopath, Christian Science practitioner or anyone else without a formal medical degree as their usual source of medical care.

Travel Time to Regular Source of Care (7)

For those who reported a regular source of care, travel time to their regular source was elicited by the question "How long does it usually take (PERSON) to get there from home, the way (he/she) usually goes?"

Appointment or Walk-In Visit to Regular Source of Care (8)

To determine if the person generally has an appointment, the following question was asked: "Does (PERSON) usually have an appointment ahead of time when (he/she) goes to (PLACE) or does (he/she) just walk in?"

Appointment Waiting Time at Regular Source of Care (9)

Those who usually have an appointment see their regular source of care were asked, "Except for emergencies, how long does (PERSON) usually have to wait to get an appointment with the doctor?"

Office Waiting Time at Regular Source of Care (10)

Respondents who indicated a regular source of care were also asked, "How long does (PERSON) usually have to wait to see the doctor, once (he/she) gets there?" This refers to the time spent waiting in the physician's office before being seen.

OUTCOME INDICES

Percent (Not) Seeing a Physician in 1970 (11)

The percent (not) seeing a physician refers to the proportion of the sample who did (or did not) have at least one physician visit during the survey year. Excluded are all persons not in the universe for all twelve months of the year.

The best estimates on this variable refer to the adjusted estimates obtained through integrating the information collected on physician visits in the social survey, with the verifications of those visits solicited from the hospitals and physicians, who purportedly rendered the services.

Mean Number of Physician Visits per Person-Year in 1970 (12)

The mean number of physician visits per person-year refers to the sum of all visits related to hospitalized illness, other nonhospitalized illness, pregnancy, other minor illness and routine checkups, shots, test, and ophthalmologist visits for the survey year. It includes seeing either a doctor or osteopath or his nurse or technician at the following sites: patient's home; doctor's office or private clinic; hospital outpatient department or emergency room; industrial, school camp or college health services; and any other clinic such as a board of health clinic or neighborhood health center. Excluded are telephone calls and visits by a doctor to a hospital inpatient.

Person-years are computed by summing the total months by sample members in the population universe during the survey year and dividing this sum by 12. The purpose of this base is to adjust for sample members who were not in the population the entire survey year, such as those who died, were institutionalized, or were born during the year.

As discussed earlier, the best estimates on this variable refer to the estimates obtained by adjusting the social survey data for the information gained from hospitals and other purported providers, on whether or not the visits did, indeed, occur.

Disability Days in Two Weeks (12)

Disability days are the sum of days reported in response to the questions: "Within the last two weeks, how many days did (PERSON) stay in bed all or part of the day because (he/she) was not feeling well?" and (apart from the days (PERSON) stayed in bed), "How many days within the last two weeks was (PERSON) not able to do the things (he/she) usually does because (he/she) was not feeling well?"

Disability days then includes bed confinement days and restricted (or reduced) activity days, when individuals limited their normal activities because of not feeling well, etc.

Physician Visits in Two Weeks (14)

The volume of physician visits in two weeks is based on the question: "When in the last two weeks did (PERSON) visit or talk on the phone to a doctor about (his/her) health?" and the follow-up question, "How many times?"

Percent of Symptoms for which Physician was Seen (15)

The respondent was given a list of symptoms and asked "Did anyone have (SYMPTOM) during 1970?" If he said yes, he was asked, "Did (PERSON) see a doctor about it during 1970 or since the first of the year?" If person said no (had *not* had the symptom in 1970), he was asked about the next symptom. If person had a symptom and did *not* see a physician for it in *1970,* he was asked, "Has (PERSON) *ever* seen a doctor about this condition or one like it?"

The 22 symptoms about which the respondents were queried were as follows: (a) cough any time during the day or night which lasted for three weeks; (b) sudden feelings of weakness or faintness; (c) getting up some mornings tired and exhausted even with a usual amount of rest; (d) feeling tired for weeks at a time for no special reason; (e) frequent headaches; (f) skin rash or breaking out on any part of the body; (g) diarrhea (loose bowel movements) for four or five days; (h) shortness of breath even after light work; (i) waking up with stiff or aching joints; (j) pains or swelling in any joint during the day; (k) frequent backaches; (l) unexplained loss of over ten pounds in weight; (m) repeated pains in or near the heart; (n) repeated indigestion or upset stomach; (o) repeated vomiting for a day or more; (p) sore throat or running nose with a fever as high as 100°F for at least two days; (q) nose stopped up, or sneezing, for two weeks or more; (r) unexpected bleeding from any part of the body not caused by accident or injury; (s) abdominal pains (pains in the belly or gut) for at least a couple of days; (t) any infections, irritations, or pains in the eyes or ears; (u) toothache; (v) bleeding gums.

The last two dental symptoms are not included in the analyses reported here, as we are primarily concerned with medically relevant symptoms.

MD Estimates of Percent of Symptoms for which Physician Should Be Seen (16)

The physicians were asked, "Of 100 people in a given age group (children 1-5, children 6-15, people 16-44, 45-65, 65 years of age or older) with each of the following (22) symptoms, please estimate what number would have a condition for which they should see a doctor." The following response categories were provided: 0-20, 21-40, 41-60, 61-80, and 81-100.

Medical Severity Index (17)

Physicians were asked to assign each diagnostic condition reported by respondents to one of the following medical severity categories: (1) preventive care or care from a physician would make no difference for this condition; (2) symptomatic relief available from a physician; (3) should see a doctor; (4) must see a doctor. Levels (1) and (2) were considered more elective health care and (3) and (4) mandatory.

The medical severity index is based on the diagnoses and visits reported by respondents in the social survey *and* on the verifications received from hospitals and physicians of whether or not the visits occurred and for what reasons (See following Medical Security Index section for further discussion of how index was constructed from social survey data, physician and hospital verifications of visits and doctor-evaluated ratings of severity).

Use-Continuity Measures (18)

The questions asked of women who had been pregnant in 1970, to elicit information on the continuity of care they received, were: "What is the name of the doctor or place that provided the *most* care for (MOTHER) during the pregnancy?" and "Which reason on this card best describes why (MOTHER) happened to go to (PHYSICIAN/PLACE) for this pregnancy?". The choices provided on the card were (1) usual doctor or clinic, (2) referred by usual doctor, (3) referred by another (not usual) doctor, (4) picked by patient or family to treat this condition, (5) recommended by other relatives or friends to treat this condition, (6) referred by someone else. Respondents were also asked at what place (person's home, doctor's office or private clinic, hospital outpatient department, hospital emergency room, industrial, school, camp or college health service, any other clinic not connected with a hospital, or in-hospital visit) the visits occurred and how many visits occurred at each location. A second question was asked with respect to "Did (MOTHER) visit any *other* doctor or clinic in connection with this pregnancy?'' Similar questions were asked, as were of the "most amount" source, with respect to the site and number of visits that occurred at this source. This line of questioning was continued until all the sources seen in connection with the pregnancy were identified.

Use of Emergency Rooms for Primary Care (19)

The head of household and spouse of head only were asked, for a selected list of medical conditions, "People react in various ways to their medical conditions. Please look at each condition and circle the number under the phrase which best describes what you would do if you had the condition." The conditions were as follows: (a) you have sharp chest pains for the first time; (b) your wrist swells two hours after a fall; (c) you have a sore throat or running nose with a fever as high as 100°F for at least two days; (d) you have your third severe headache in as many days; (e) you cut your finger deeply with a dirty knife.

The alternatives provided, with respect to what the persons might do were: (1) call ambulance at once; (2) go to hospital emergency room same day; (3) see my doctor within three days; (4) see my doctor within one month; (5) do nothing (treat it myself).

The same panel of physicians, who were asked to evaluate the number of people out of 100 with a specific symptom who should see a doctor for that symptom (See following Symptoms-Response Ratio section), were also asked to indicate, for certain age groups (under 35, 35-64, 65 and over), which was the "medically appropriate response" to these five conditions. For three of the conditions — chest pains, swollen wrist, and cutting finger with a dirty knife — they recommended that people in all age groups, go to a hospital emergency room (or, in the case of people 65 and over, call an ambulance for chest pains). For the remaining two — sore throat with fever and severe headaches — they suggested that people in all three age groups see the doctor within two days (See later discussion for more detailed description of how these physician ratings were obtained).

Satisfaction (20)

The head of household and spouse of head only were asked, "Thinking over the medical care you and those close to you have received over the past few years from doctors and hospitals, how satisfied have you been with each of the following: (list of items). They were asked to indicate whether they were "very satisfied," "satisfied," "unsatisfied," or "very dissatisfied."

The items were (a) overall quality of the medical care received; (b) waiting time in doctor's office or clinics; (c) availability of medical care at night and the weekends; (d) ease and convenience of getting to a doctor from where you live; (e) the out-of-pocket costs of the medical care received; (f) the information given to you about what you should do at home to treat illness; (h) the courtesy and consideration shown you by doctors; (i) the courtesy and consideration shown by nurses; (j) the follow-up care received after an initial treatment or operation; (k) concern of doctors for your overall health rather than just for an isolated symptom or disease; (l) getting all your medical needs taken care of at one location; (m) information you have been able to obtain to help you choose a physician.

Symptoms-Response Ratio

DETERMINATION OF PHYSICIAN ESTIMATES

Forty doctors from the teaching faculty of the University of Chicago Pritzker School of Medicine were given a questionnaire listing the 22 symptoms found in the 1970 Center for Health Administration Studies questionnaire in the summer of 1970 (See previous Definition of Variables section). These physicians were distributed as follows with respect to their faculty tenure and specialty:

Tenure		Specialty	
Instructor	4	Internist	13
Asst. Prof.	14	Surgeon	9
Assoc. Prof.	13	OB/GYN	6
Professor	9	Pediatrics	7
		Psychiatry	5
	40		40

Each doctor was asked to estimate, based on his training and experience, how many people out of 100 manifesting a certain symptom should see a doctor for it. The number was estimated in terms of five general categories: 0-20, 21-40, 41-60, 61-80, 81-100. Furthermore, the ratings for each symptom were obtained separately for each of the five following categories of patients: 1-5, 6-15, 16-44, 45-65, and 65 and over.

To determine the number of a given age group with a specified symptom who should see a physician for it, the mid-point[1] of the response category chosen by each physician for each age-symptom complex was

---

[1]For example, if the response category for a particular age-symptom complex was 41-60, the mid-point used for averaging was 50.

summed for all the physicians responding, and divided by the number of responses. Table 28 shows what the resulting mean physician ratings are for the various age-symptom complexes.

Two aspects of the reliability of these physicians' ratings that may be evaluated are the inter-rater (the level of agreement *between* physicians) and intra-rater (the consistency of ratings by the *same* physician at different points in time) reliability of the estimates.

A Chi-square goodness of fit test was conducted on the distribution of physician responses to the question about the number of people out of 100 in a certain age group with a given symptom who should see a doctor for that symptom. The number of physicians who chose each of the response categories (0-20, 21-40, 41-60, etc.) for each age-symptom

TABLE 28

Mean physician ratings[a] of number of people out of 100 (percent) with selected symptoms in particular age groups who should see a doctor for that symptom

	MEAN NUMBER OF PEOPLE OUT OF 100 (PERCENT) WITH SYMPTOM WHO SHOULD SEE DOCTOR, BY AGE GROUPS				
SYMPTOM	1-5	6-15	16-44	45-64	65+
Cough	53.2	52.1	52.5	61.0	65.5
Weakness	45.9	45.3	51.0	61.5	62.5
Tired mornings	41.5	38.6	37.2	41.0	43.0
Tired for weeks	59.1	53.2	46.0	50.0	46.0
Headaches	61.5	54.2	47.0	47.5	52.5
Rash	43.7	39.5	39.2	41.8	41.5
Diarrhea	48.9	42.1	40.0	46.0	48.5
Shortness of breath	83.1	77.6	71.0	74.5	72.6
Aching joints	64.5	60.5	53.5	50.0	44.5
Pain or swelling in joints	71.1	71.1	60.5	60.0	55.5
Backaches	58.0	50.5	41.0	39.0	37.5
Weight loss	82.9	77.0	73.5	74.6	78.0
Heart pains	59.0	53.7	66.5	72.5	76.5
Indigestion	49.4	40.0	51.5	50.5	56.2
Vomiting	59.2	51.1	55.0	54.5	62.0
Sore throat	42.6	40.0	36.0	36.0	39.0
Sneezing	34.7	30.5	28.0	26.5	30.0
Bleeding	82.4	77.4	80.5	82.5	84.0
Pains in the gut	64.3	60.0	60.5	60.5	64.5
Infected eyes or ears	60.9	61.4	52.6	53.6	55.1

[a]To determine these mean physician ratings, the mid-point of the response category chosen by each physician for each age-symptom complex was summed for all the physicians responding, and divided by the number of responses. The respective categories (and their mid-points) are as follows: 0-20 (10); 21-40 (30); 41-60 (50); 61-80 (70); and 81-100 (90).

complex was compared with the number of physicians who would fall in each category, if their responses were evenly distributed among each of the five categories. For example, if there were 40 physician raters and no consensus among them as to how many in a given age-symptom complex should go see a doctor, then their responses might be expected to be evenly distributed among the five categories, with eight doctors responding to each of the five "number-who-should go" groupings. This is the type of theoretical distribution against which the actual distribution of physician responses were compared, to calculate the Chi-square goodness of fit test of inter-rater reliability.

Table 29 shows (1) the mid-point of the modal category of physician ratings of the number of patients in a given age-symptom complex who should see a doctor for that symptom and (2) whether the overall distribution of physician responses in the various categories is statistically different from a theoretically random one.

In general, the level of consensus among physicians varies, depending on the age and symptom considered. There appears to be more agreement among physicians with respect to the percent of the older age categories who should see a doctor for symptoms. Also, there is greater consensus when considering the most severe (shortness of breath, pain or swelling in joints, weight loss, sudden bleeding) and least severe (sore throat, sneezing) symptoms.

An analysis of variations in physician ratings by specialty and faculty tenure suggested that obstetrician-gynecologists, psychiatrists and instructors tended to assign the highest severity ratings to symptoms and pediatricians and full professors, respectively, the lowest.

To test the intra-rater reliability of physician ratings, a subsample of 15 of the 40 original physician raters were re-interviewed within six weeks and asked to respond to the same questions regarding the percent of people of a certain age-symptom complex who should see a doctor.

Pearson and Kendall correlation coefficients were computed on the test and retest ratings given by physicians. The findings from the Pearson and Kendall correlation analyses were quite similar. The Pearson correlation coefficients are reported here (See Table 30).

In general, there were statistically significant test-retest correlation coefficients for each of the age-symptom complexes, although considerable variation is evident in physician rankings over time. The lowest correlations were found for the least severe conditions.

TABLE 29
Mid-point of modal category of physician ratings [a] of number of people out of 100 (percent) with selected symptoms in particular age groups who should see a doctor for that symptom

	MID-POINT OF MODAL CATEGORY OF MD RATINGS OF NUMBER OF PEOPLE OUT OF 100 (PERCENT) WITH SYMPTOM WHO SHOULD SEE DOCTOR, BY AGE GROUPS				
SYMPTOM	1-5	6-15	16-44	45-64	65+
Cough	90	50	70	30	90*
Weakness	10	30	50	50,70*[b]	70*
Tired mornings	10	10*	10	10	50
Tired for weeks	70	70	30,50[b]	50	50
Headaches	90	70	70	50	30
Rash	30	50	10	30,50[b]	50
Diarrhea	50	30	30,50[b]	30	50
Shortness of breath	90**	90**	90**	90**	90**
Aching joints	90*	90	50	30,70[b]	10
Pain or swelling in joints	90**	90**	90*	90	90
Backache	50	50	50*	30*	10*
Weight loss	90**	90**	90**	90**	90**
Heart pains	90	70	90*	90**	90**
Indigestion	50	50*	40*	50*	50,70*[b]
Vomiting	90	70	30,70[b]	70	70
Sore throat	10	10	10*	10*	30
Sneezing	10,30*[b]	30**	10**	10**	10,30**[b]
Bleeding	90**	90**	90**	90**	90**
Pains in the gut	90	90	90*	50*	50**
Infected eyes or ears	90	90	30,90[b]	30	30

*Distribution for which this is the mid-point of the modal category varied significantly at (P ≤ .05), using Chi-square test, from hypothetical distribution in which responses are randomly allocated to each of the five categories.

**Distribution for which this is the mid-point of the modal category varied significantly at (P ≤ .001), using Chi-square test, from hypothetical distribution in which responses are randomly allocated to each of the five categories.

[a] The response categories (and their mid-points) are as follows: 0-20 (10); 21-40 (30); 41-60 (50); 61-80 (70); 81-100 (90).

[b] There were two modal categories of physician ratings for this age-symptom complex.

TABLE 30
Test-retest Pearson correlation coefficients of physician ratings of symptoms by age groups

SYMPTOM	PEARSON CORRELATION COEFFICIENTS, BY AGE GROUPS				
	1-5	6-15	16-44	45-64	65+
Cough	.49*	.35	.38	.39	.12
Weakness	.80**	.73*	.37	.41	.47*
Tired mornings	−.02	.48*	.57*	.68*	.41
Tired for weeks	−.32	.26	.18	.38	.59*
Headaches	.38	.20	.38	.56*	.62*
Rash	.76**	.73**	.75**	.85**	.81**
Diarrhea	.83**	.86**	.66*	.74**	.53*
Shortness of breath	.11	.57*	.61*	.15	.32
Aching joints	−.06	.19	.49*	.61*	.86**
Pain or swelling in joints	.59*	.28	.69*	.55*	.73**
Backaches	.47	.25	.24	.57*	.38
Weight loss	.87**	.76**	.79*	.61*	.45*
Heart pains	.73*	.14	.19	.16	.22
Indigestion	.22	.35	.60*	.51*	.44
Vomiting	.69*	.80**	.62*	.71**	.41
Sore throat	.15	.34	.58*	.53*	.47*
Sneezing	.39	.80**	.33	.51*	.58*
Bleeding	.75**	.88**	.82**	.54*	.56*
Pains in the gut	.56*	.80**	.48*	.59*	.59*
Infected eyes or ears	.78**	.90**	.69*	.46*	.51*

*Significant (P ≤ .05).
**Significant (P ≤ .001).

DETERMINATION OF COMPUTATIONAL FORMULA[2]

Table 31 provides a hypothetical example of how the symptoms-response ratio is computed. In essence, the ratio describes the extent to which the actual number of visits to a doctor in response to symptoms, is greater than, equal to or less than the number that the panel of physicians estimate should occur.

Part A of Table 31 describes a hypothetical example of how many people in certain age groups in a population may experience selected symptoms. Part B shows how the actual and expected number of visits for a population with this particular mix and symptoms might be computed in terms of the percent who should and do go to a doctor for the

[2]The computational formula used in this report differs from one used in a Preliminary Report on this study, entitled, "Development of a Framework for the Study of Access to

symptoms. Part C, which is mathematically equivalent to the procedure used in B, simply points out that the actual and expected number of visits may be attached to each individual in a given age-symptom complex and summed, to produce the respective components of the symptoms-response ratio.

DETERMINATION OF TEST OF SIGNIFICANCE

The computational formula for the symptoms-response ratio,

$\dfrac{A-E}{E}$, approximates that of a Chi-square test statistic

$\sum \dfrac{(0-E)^2}{E}$ where 0 = observed frequencies and E = expected frequencies in the cells of a contingency table.

The following statistic, based on the formula for the symptoms-response index and the Chi-square statistic, was computed for each population subgroup reported in Table 16, and compared with the values in a Chi-square Distribution table (degrees of freedom = 1), to see if the difference between the actual and expected values in the ratio differed significantly from chance for each group:

$$\dfrac{(A-E)^2}{E}$$

Health Care," by L. A. Aday, et al., Center for Health Administration Studies, University of Chicago (October, 1973).

The formula used in that publication was as follows:

$$\sum_{a=1}^{22} \left[\left(\dfrac{\text{proportion of people with symptom "a" who see a doctor}}{\text{proportion of people with symptom "a" who physicians estimate should see a doctor}} - 1.00 \right) \left(\text{proportion symptom "a" represents of total mix of symptoms} \right) \right]$$

The new formula offers the following advantages over this formula: (1) it sums the actual and expected visits for each symptom *before* dividing to get the ratio (ratio of sums), which reduces the random variation in the index, compared to the old formula, which divided the actual by expected number of visits for *each* symptom and *then* summed across all the symptoms (sums of ratios); (2) the components of the new formula are self-weighting, i.e., the actual and expected values both depend on the number of symptoms experienced; (3) it permits the actual and estimated number of visits for each individual in the sample to be determined (see Table 31); (4) it is easier to compute; (5) it is more readily interpretable, as the degree to which the actual number of visits in response to symptoms of illness is greater than, equal to, or less than the number a panel of medical experts would suggest; and (6) unlike the computations for the original formula, the findings reported here for the symptoms-response ratio include only the *medically*-relevant symptoms evaluated by physicians, i.e., the dental symptoms are excluded.

TABLE 31

Explanation of formula for computing symptoms-response ratio

A. Hypothetical example

SYMPTOM	A_1	AGE GROUPS A_2	A_3	A_4	A_5
. S_1	$n_{1,1}{}^a = 4$	$n_{1,2} = 5$			
S_2	$n_{2,1} = 6$				
S_3	$n_{3,1} = 0$				
S_{22}					

B. Ratio expressed as *percentage* of individuals in age-symptom complex

1) No. out of 100 (%) in given age-symptom complex who *do* see doctor (A)

$$25\% \text{ of } n_{1,1}(4) = 1.00$$
$$60\% \text{ of } n_{1,2}(5) = 3.00$$
$$33\% \text{ of } n_{2,1}(6) = 2.00$$
$$\underline{\quad} = \underline{\quad}$$
$$6.00$$

2) MD est. of no. out of 100 (%) in given age-symptom complex who *should* see doctor (E)

$$40\% \text{ of } n_{1,1}(4) = 1.60$$
$$55\% \text{ of } n_{1,2}(5) = 2.75$$
$$60\% \text{ of } n_{2,1}(6) = 3.60$$
$$80\% \text{ of } n_{3,1}(0) = \underline{\quad}$$
$$7.95$$

3) Symptoms-response ratio $= \dfrac{(A-E)\,(100)}{E} = \dfrac{(6.00-7.95)\,(100)}{7.95} = -24.53$

C. Ratio expressed as *values for* individuals in age-symptom complex

	1) Whether or not individual in given age-symptom complex *does see* doctor(A)[b]	2) MD est. of whether or not individual in given age-symptom complex *should see* doctor (E)[c]
	(A)	(E)
	1	.4
individuals in group	0	.4
$n_{1,1}$	0	.4
	0	.4
	1	.55
	1	.55
individuals in group	1	.55
$n_{1,2}$	0	.55
	0	.55
	1	.6
	1	.6
individuals in group	0	.6
$n_{2,1}$	0	.6
	0	.6
individuals in group	0	0
$n_{3,1}$		
	6.00	7.95

3) Symptoms-response ratio $= \dfrac{(A-E)\,(100)}{E} = \dfrac{(6.00-7.95)\,(100)}{7.95} = -24.53$

[a]$n_{i,j}$ = no. of people with symptom i in age group j.

[b]1 = person with symptom saw doctor

0 = person with symptom *did not* see doctor or person did not have symptom

[c]These are based on MD est., expressed as decimals. If person did not experience the symptom, the MD est. equals 0.

Prior to computing the test statistic itself, the actual and estimated number of visits for each symptom for each subgroup were divided by the mean sample weight for that subgroup. This procedure serves to reduce values on the test statistic, inflated by the sample weighting factors. As such, it tends to make the significance test more conservative, i.e., it is more difficult to reject the null hypothesis that there is no difference between the actual and expected values in the ratio, because the magnitude of the test statistic becomes smaller.

Expanding the symptoms-response computational formula to a Chi-square-type test statistic, and adjusting it for the influence of weighting factors does, the authors believe, enhance the potential usefulness of the index for testing the statistical significance of the differences between the number of visits there are and the number of visits there should be, according to M.D. judgments, in response to symptoms of illness in a population.

Medical Severity Index[3]

The approach used in constructing the medical severity index has combined the use of the I.C.D.A. classification scheme with a method of physician-determined evaluations of medical severity.

The I.C.D.A. index was used as a starting point and was summarized into approximately 70 categories which seemed appropriate as reasons for seeing a physician. Ten more categories were added, for such items as check-ups, birth control advice, and minor social and emotional problems seen by non-psychiatrists. These categories were then used to code the first 100 families of the 4,000 sampled in the 1970 CHAS study. The coding was done by two social science graduate students and a medical student and then by a board-certified internist. On the basis of this coding, about ten new categories were added, other categories were rearranged, and an agreement was made for the coders to hold all cases for the internist which they could not agree upon among themselves or which they could not locate in a standard physician's diagnostic text. About 10 percent of all diagnoses were held for the internist.

The medical consultants and coders agreed that a more detailed set of codes could be used for coding diagnoses provided by hospitals and

---

[3]This discussion of the medical severity index is based on an article, entitled "Health Care Need and Actual Use by Age, Race, and Income," currently being written by the designers of the index — Joanna Kravits, Research Associate, Center for Health Administration Studies, University of Chicago and John Schneider, M.D., Asst. Professor, Department of Medicine, Billings Hospital, University of Chicago.

physicians. For example, "heart trouble" excluded "heart attack" (acute myocardial infarction) and "heart failure," both of which had their own individual codes, but still included a variety of diagnoses ranging from trivial to serious. In addition, there was a category of uncodable diagnoses which accounted for about one percent of all diagnoses given.

The medical consultant and staff modified the diagnostic codes before going to physicians and hospitals to verify the diagnoses and visits reported by respondents in the social survey. The codes were enlarged from two digits to three digits so that sub-categories could be added to those codes such as heart trouble in which medical professionals could be expected to give more accurate diagnoses than the respondents, and several new categories were developed. In analyzing the data, the diagnoses from the verifications always took precedence over the diagnoses from the social survey.

Positive verifications of the diagnoses and visits were obtained for 58 percent of physician contacts and for 83 percent of hospital stays, including new hospital stays and physician contacts which had not been mentioned by the respondent. Negative verifications, which confirmed that the patient had reported care which had not occurred in 1970, accounted for an additional ten percent of physician contacts and eight percent of hospital stays. This care was eliminated from analysis of the utilization data. Adjusting for eliminated care and care new to the verifications, the overall completion rate for which diagnoses were available from the verifications was 93 percent for hospital stays and 68 percent for physician care. In other words, only seven percent of diagnoses for hospital stays and 32 percent for physician care had to be taken from the respondent's reporting of diagnoses in the social survey, rather than from the M.D. verifications of these visits and diagnoses.

While useful for many types of analyses, the diagnostic codes do not by themselves provide an estimate of the medical necessity of the care given. In order to do this, a four part rating scheme was set up:

1 = preventive care or care from a physician would make no difference for this condition
2 = symptomatic relief available from physician
3 = should see a doctor
4 = must see a doctor

The rating was performed by a panel of five M.D.'s — two internists, a psychiatrist, a psychiatrist with a secondary specialty in internal medicine, and a recent medical school graduate. Using this rating scheme, total agreement on severity was reached on 24 percent of the diagnoses given by the respondents and also on 24 percent of the much more finely divided diagnoses given by physicians and hospitals. A difference in severity ratings of one in either direction was achieved in an additional 75 percent of respondent diagnoses and 66 percent of professional diagnoses.

This procedure left one percent of the respondent diagnoses (which happened to be only one category — blindness) and ten percent of the professional diagnoses with differences of M.D. opinion of more than one point on the scaling. The one respondent category (blindness) was eliminated from the analysis and the professional verifications in which there were disagreements were resolved by assigning the severity code based upon the two digit diagnostic code in the social survey. The mode of the five physicians' ratings was taken in each case.

It is obvious from the above discussion that a given individual can have more than one diagnosis and therefore more than one severity code on the 1 to 4 point scale. Various ways were considered of combining these diagnoses to arrive at a summary of the severity of illness for which the patient sought medical care in 1970. It seemed logical that when a physician was seen for both severe and trivial conditions, this was a different case than either being seen for a trivial or preventive care only or for care of a serious illness only. From this conclusion, evolved a three point summary scale of all of the severity codes for a given individual's doctor contacts during the year:

A = elective care only (modal categories of severity code for all diagnoses are 1 or 2)

B = both elective and mandatory care (modal categories are 1 through 4)

C = mandatory care only (modal categories of severity codes for all diagnoses are 3 or 4)

This scaling does have several drawbacks. Obviously, it works best for the two-thirds of the population who consult a physician during the year on an outpatient basis and who have complaints spread over the entire spectrum of illness from trivial to fatal. It works much less well for hospitalized patients, whose illnesses can be assumed to be usually mandatory in the sense of requiring physician care. And it does not apply at all to the one-third of the population who did not see a doctor during the year.

Use of Emergency Rooms for Primary Care

As described in the first section of Chapter 3, heads of households and the wife of the head were asked to indicate for five medical conditions, what action they were apt to take in response to these conditions — call an ambulance, go to a hospital emergency room, see their doctor within two days, etc.

The same panel of physicians who were asked to assign severity ratings to the symptoms incorporated in the symptoms-response ratio, were also queried about what would be the "medically appropriate response" to these five conditions for certain age groups (under 35, 35-64, 65 and over).

Table 32 shows what the modal response category was for the 40 physician raters and whether they were statistically different from a theoretically random distribution.[4] These modal categories were taken as the responses deemed to be most "medically appropriate." For each of the age-condition complexes, the distribution of physician responses was statistically different from a theoretically random one (p ≤ .001). The physician evaluations of the "medically appropriate response" to these conditions, then, may be considered statistically reliable estimates.

Sample Design[5]

The universe sampled in this study was the total, non-institutionalized population of the United States. This universe excludes the following individuals:

1) residents in medical, mental, penal, religious, or other institutions who were not residents of a private dwelling at any time during 1970;

2) residents on military reservations (the latter three studies included, however, personnel in the armed forces living off base with their families or in other civilian households); and

3) transient individuals having no usual or permanent residence.

---

[4]The Chi-square goodness fit test was used to determine whether the physician responses departed from a theoretically random distribution. This theoretical distribution was constructed in the same way as the one used to test the interrater reliability of the symptom-severity ratings (See the Symptoms-Response Ratio section of this chapter).

[5]This description of the sample design is based on a discussion that appears in *Health Service Use: National Trends and Variations – 1953-1971* by R. Andersen, et al., Washington: National Center for Health Services Research and Development, U.S. Dept. HEW Publication No. (HSM) 73-3004, 1972, pp. 43-44; 49-51.

TABLE 32
Modal category of physician ratings of appropriate response to selected conditions by age groups

	MODAL CATEGORY OF MD RATINGS OF APPROPRIATE RESPONSE[a] TO CONDITION, BY AGE GROUPS		
CONDITION	Under 35	35-64	65+
Sharp chest pains	2**	2**	1 and 2**[b]
Wrist swells after fall	2**	2**	2**
Sore throat and running fever	3**	3**	3**
Third headache in three days	3**	3**	3**
Cut finger with dirty knife	2**	2**	2**

**Distribution for which this is the modal category varied significantly at (P ≤ .001), using Chi-square test, from hypothetical distribution in which responses are randomly allocated to each of the five categories.

[a]The five categories, from which physicians were asked to select the "medically appropriate response" were as follows: 1) call ambulance at once; 2) go to hospital emergency room same day; 3) see my doctor within three days; 4) see my doctor within one month; 5) do nothing (treat it myself).

[b]There were two modal categories of physician ratings for this age-condition complex.

The NORC master sample used in this study is essentially the same as that used in the 1964 study. Since details concerning this sample have been published in the final report for the previous study, the description here will be limited to the special characteristics of the sample design for the 1971 study (Andersen and Anderson, 1967).

The sample in the current study was not a self-weighting area probability sample of the U.S. population. Rather it overrepresented people of special concern in health policy formulation including those with low incomes living in central cities, the rural population, and persons 66 and over.

In order to obtain a sample with these special characteristics, four separate subsamples were drawn:

1) a sample (U) selected from 73 special urban segments in the NORC master sample. These segments were so designated because of the presence of a high proportion of low income urban families according to 1960 Census data;

2) a sample (A) selected from the remaining segments in the NORC national probability sample;

3) a sample (S) consisting of families either classified as low income or containing a person 66 years or older obtained by screening households in all NORC segments;[6] and

4) a sample (R) obtained from 30 additional rural primary sampling units drawn especially for this study. Only families thought to be living in rural areas of these PSU's were interviewed. No screening procedure was involved for this sample.

Table 33 shows the completion rates for each of the subsamples in the study. The estimates in the report are based on those families which were interviewed. The amount of discrepancy between these estimates and the figures which would have been obtained with full response depends, for any characteristic being estimated, on how different the non-interview families were with respect to this characteristic from those who were interviewed. It would probably be safe to assume in most cases a bias due to nonresponse of not more than 3½ percentage points. This error would appear if the interview cases split 50-50 on the item being measured and those not interviewed split 30-70.

Given the complex sampling design of this study, a weighting scheme was applied before estimates and tabulations could be produced. Weighting was necessary to correct for the different probabilities of selection among sample observations. Adjustment was also made for the varying completion rates among the various subsamples. A final post-stratification adjustment in the weights was employed to make the sample more closely representative of the actual U.S. population and thus reduce sampling variance. The control factor is the ratio of estimates from the *Current Population Survey*[7] to estimates based on the NORC sample for some 16 population classes defined by family size, family income, race and whether or not the family dwelling unit is in a Standard Metropolitan Statistical Area.

---

[6]See the Definitions of Variables section for description of "low income" (below poverty level) families.

[7]*Current Population Reports,* Series P-60, No. 80, October 4, 1971, pp. 30-32.

TABLE 33
Final completion rates

SAMPLE	ORIG.[b] ASS.	VAC/[c] NDU	WR[e]	NQ[f]	EXTRA[g] FU	NET[h] ASS.	CC[i]	COMP.[j] RATE	FINAL[k] NIR
A	1515	176	5	d	42	1376	1119	.813	257
S_1[a]	2887	407	9	d	68	2539	2451	.965	88
S_2[a]	2451	d	d	1539	d	912	785	.861	127
U	2068	415	43	d	72	1682	1378	.819	304
R	810	126	d	d	15	699	601	.859	98

[a]The report on the S sample is divided into two parts. S_1 refers to the screening operation. S_2 refers to the regular interviewing.
[b]Number of dwelling units listed in the original sampling frame.
[c]Dwelling units which were vacant during the interviewing period or had been torn down between the time of listing and the time of interviewing.
[d]Not applicable.
[e]Indicates wrong race. Some urban segments in the NORC master sample are stratified according to race. When a respondent of the wrong race was observed, no interview was conducted in that household.
[f]Indicates not qualified. Applicable only in the S sample where families were screened out if they were non-poor and had no member 66 or over.
[g]Indicates extra family units. These units were added when multiple family dwelling units were discovered at the time of interview or multiple dwelling units within the same structure had originally been listed as single units.
[h]Net assignment is equal to b-c-e-f-g.
[i]Indicates number of completed interviews.
[j]Completion rate is equal to i/h.
[k]Non-interview reports include "refusals," "breakoffs," "no one home after repeated calls," "language problems," "respondent too ill to be interviewed," etc.

4

Review of the Literature

Introduction

This section describes the literature that was reviewed in the process of formulating the access concept.

This report on the literature review is divided into three parts: 1) a key to the literature on the access concept (in terms of the framework); 2) the bibliography and list of references themselves; and 3) selected abstracts relevant to important theoretical or empirical issues of access.

The key (or index) to the literature is presented in outline form in terms of "access" itself as a concept, important process and outcome indicators of access and methodological issues relevant to the measurement and prediction of the concept. The numbers in parentheses after each section of the outline refer to references in the bibliography that include information on these topics.

The bibliography contains the list of references reviewed, in alphabetical order. Identifying numbers are assigned, in sequence, to each citation.

References that provide data on the behavior of potential process and outcome indices of access were summarized. These abstracts serve to update a bibliography on the indices and correlates of health services utilization,[1] published in early 1972. These abstracts report the purpose, population and/or sample and method of data collection, process and outcome indices of access, method of data analysis and findings for each reference. The emphasis was on abstracting *empirical* articles on the access concept. Some few theoretical books and articles are also included, however.[2]

Key to the Literature on the Access Concept

I.   "ACCESS" AS A CONCEPT

      (16, 22, 54, 58, 66, 76, 91, 92, 119, 121, 131, 157, 178, 205, 225, 350, 385, 394, 403, 406, 411)

II.   PROCESS INDICES

      A. *Characteristics of Health Delivery System*

         1. Resources

            a. Volume

               (8, 16, 22, 26, 32, 37, 59, 66, 76, 82, 90, 91, 92, 96, 109, 112, 115, 119, 121, 125, 129, 130, 131, 139, 149, 178, 213, 226, 235, 281, 311, 312, 325, 327, 348, 349, 350, 371, 377, 394, 395, 406)

            b. Distribution

               (8, 16, 22, 26, 32, 37, 59, 66, 76, 82, 90, 91, 92, 96, 109, 112, 115, 119, 121, 125, 129, 130, 131, 149, 159, 178,

---

[1]The following references are abstracted in *The Utilization of Health Services: Indices and Correlates —A Research Bibliography* by L. A. Aday and R. L. Eichhorn, Washington: National Center for Health Services Research and Development, U.S. Department HEW Publication No. (HSM) 73-3003, 1972, in a format similar to the one used here: 2, 4, 9, 10, 11, 13, 14, 15, 17, 18, 19, 20, 23, 24, 29, 32, 36, 38, 40, 41, 42, 43, 45, 47, 50, 51, 52, 57, 60, 62, 63, 64, 65, 69, 73, 74, 77, 78, 79, 81, 83, 84, 85, 86, 87, 88, 89, 93, 96, 100, 105, 109, 110, 111, 114, 115, 120, 122, 123, 126, 133, 135, 136, 138, 140, 141, 143, 144, 148, 165, 171, 172, 173, 179, 180, 181, 182, 184, 186, 188, 189, 193, 194, 195, 196, 197, 198, 201, 203, 204, 205, 210, 211, 221, 222, 224, 240, 241 thru 265, 279 thru 287, 292 thru 297, 304, 305, 308, 310, 313, 315, 317, 318, 321, 322, 323, 324, 326, 328, 330, 332, 334, 335, 337, 340, 341, 344, 346, 347, 348, 349, 351, 352, 353, 355, 356, 357, 358, 359, 360, 361, 372, 376, 377, 378, 379, 381, 382, 387, 390, 395, 397, 400, 401, 402, 405, 408, 409, 410, 411, 414, 417, 418, 420, 421, 423, 424, 427, 429, 430, 431.

[2]These abstracts are contained in the Research Appendix, Chapter 5.

213, 219, 226, 235, 281, 311, 312, 325, 327, 350, 371, 394, 395, 406)

2. Organization

a. Entry

(3, 16, 22, 37, 48, 50, 56, 66, 76, 82, 90, 91, 92, 112, 115, 121, 125, 129, 130, 213, 309, 312, 327, 350, 379, 388, 394, 417, 418)

b. Structure

(11, 13, 16, 20, 22, 23, 24, 36, 37, 40, 54, 56, 62, 66, 70, 76, 82, 83, 86, 87, 90, 91, 92, 102, 109, 112, 115, 121, 125, 129, 130, 135, 136, 138, 139, 145, 148, 156, 159, 165, 166, 167, 183, 185, 186, 188, 195, 203, 213, 219, 220, 223, 226, 235, 281, 282, 283, 284, 287, 288, 289, 290, 291, 292, 293, 294, 295, 296, 297, 298, 299, 302, 303, 308, 310, 312, 317, 318, 320, 324, 325, 327, 330, 332, 334, 335, 343, 346, 347, 350, 352, 365, 374, 375, 376, 381, 382, 384, 386, 394, 395, 396, 401, 409, 412, 423, 428)

B. *Characteristics of Population-at-Risk*

1. Predisposing

a. Mutable

1) General health care beliefs and attitudes

(4, 13, 17, 22, 25, 35, 36, 37, 45, 55, 56, 58, 60, 62, 64, 65, 77, 78, 79, 92, 101, 104, 108, 114, 120, 126, 130, 141, 144, 150, 155, 159, 163, 167, 175, 179, 180, 181, 182, 184, 196, 197, 198, 206, 211, 213, 218, 222, 229, 312, 314, 322, 323, 324, 327, 328, 355, 356, 357, 363, 364, 372, 387, 400, 402, 403, 408, 414, 419, 426, 431, 432)

2) Knowledge and sources of health care information

(17, 22, 36, 45, 55, 56, 69, 77, 84, 92, 93, 104, 108, 133, 155, 167, 175, 197, 198, 206, 213, 324, 355, 372, 387)

3) Stress and anxiety about health

(9, 10, 22, 45, 51, 52, 55, 64, 71, 73, 98, 104, 114, 126,
163, 179, 180, 181, 182, 197, 198, 211, 213, 221, 222,
229, 314, 323, 324, 327, 341, 355, 356, 357, 363, 364,
408, 424, 429)

b. Immutable

1) Age

(3, 4, 5, 15, 17, 18, 19, 21, 22, 23, 24, 25, 26, 27, 32,
35, 36, 37, 38, 41, 42, 43, 47, 51, 52, 55, 57, 62, 64, 65,
67, 73, 81, 83, 85, 86, 87, 92, 98, 100, 101, 103, 104,
108, 109, 110, 113, 114, 115, 121, 123, 125, 130, 142,
144, 145, 146, 150, 151, 152, 153, 154, 155, 157, 158,
163, 166, 167, 172, 173, 184, 189, 203, 205, 209, 210,
213, 218, 220, 222, 226, 229, 240, 241, 242, 243, 244,
245, 246, 247, 248, 249, 250, 252, 253, 255, 256, 257,
258, 259, 260, 261, 262, 263, 264, 265, 266, 267, 268,
269, 270, 271, 272, 273, 274, 275, 276, 277, 278, 279,
280, 282, 283, 284, 285, 286, 287, 288, 290, 291, 292,
293, 294, 295, 296, 297, 298, 299, 300, 301, 302, 303,
304, 305, 307, 310, 311, 313, 314, 315, 320, 322, 323,
325, 326, 327, 335, 337, 340, 342, 359, 361, 363, 372,
375, 378, 390, 396, 402, 403, 406, 409, 410, 412, 415,
416, 417, 418, 419, 420, 425, 426, 427, 428)

2) Sex

(3, 5, 17, 18, 21, 22, 23, 24, 26, 27, 35, 36, 37, 38, 41,
43, 47, 62, 65, 67, 83, 85, 86, 87, 92, 103, 104, 108,
109, 110, 113, 114, 115, 117, 121, 130, 142, 144, 145,
146, 157, 158, 163, 167, 172, 173, 184, 203, 205, 209,
213, 220, 223, 240, 241, 242, 243, 244, 245, 246, 247,
248, 249, 250, 252, 253, 255, 256, 257, 258, 259, 260,
262, 263, 264, 265, 266, 267, 268, 269, 270, 271, 272,
273, 274, 275, 276, 277, 278, 279, 280, 282, 283, 284,
285, 286, 287, 288, 290, 291, 292, 293, 294, 295, 296,
297, 298, 299, 300, 301, 302, 303, 307, 310, 311, 314,
315, 320, 325, 326, 327, 342, 359, 372, 375, 378, 390,
402, 403, 409, 410, 415, 416, 417, 418, 419, 426, 427,
428)

3) Marital status

(17, 22, 23, 24, 35, 47, 55, 81, 109, 110, 113, 114, 115,
124, 130, 142, 144, 157, 158, 172, 205, 220, 222, 228,
229, 244, 245, 246, 248, 250, 258, 295, 267, 271, 276,
286, 290, 292, 293, 294, 295, 296, 302, 314, 320, 327,
335, 337, 415, 416, 424)

4) Previous health behavior

(4, 17, 19, 22, 47, 62, 67, 84, 93, 101, 111, 114, 122,
124, 130, 133, 146, 162, 167, 181, 184, 197, 198, 213,
222, 229, 256, 304, 305, 322, 323, 327, 355, 360, 414,
415, 425, 426, 431)

5) Education

(1, 2, 3, 4, 5, 17, 18, 19, 22, 23, 24, 32, 36, 37, 50, 52,
55, 60, 65, 73, 74, 77, 81, 83, 84, 89, 92, 93, 100, 101,
108, 109, 110, 114, 115, 122, 130, 142, 150, 151, 152,
153, 154, 155, 157, 158, 162, 172, 181, 197, 202, 205,
210, 213, 220, 221, 222, 228, 244, 245, 247, 248, 294,
250, 253, 258, 260, 261, 267, 273, 274, 278, 304, 307,
314, 322, 323, 324, 327, 335, 342, 344, 355, 359, 361,
372, 373, 385, 399, 400, 403, 409, 415, 416, 419, 425,
426, 431)

6) Race or ethnicity

(1, 2, 3, 5, 12, 17, 18, 19, 21, 22, 24, 25, 26, 27, 29, 32,
37, 50, 51, 52, 58, 65, 67, 71, 73, 74, 81, 89, 92, 101,
103, 104, 114, 117, 121, 130, 139, 142, 144, 150, 157,
158, 162, 163, 174, 202, 205, 206, 209, 210, 213, 218,
221, 222, 244, 245, 248, 249, 250, 253, 258, 261, 262,
264, 266, 267, 268, 269, 271, 273, 274, 276, 278, 279,
280, 288, 290, 292, 293, 294, 295, 296, 298, 299, 301,
302, 303, 304, 305, 307, 310, 322, 323, 340, 342, 344,
355, 361, 372, 373, 385, 390, 403, 405, 406, 409, 410,
415, 416, 419, 425, 431, 432)

7) Family size and composition

(1, 3, 4, 12, 17, 19, 22, 24, 47, 48, 52, 55, 73, 81, 85,
92, 109, 110, 113, 142, 145, 146, 157, 162, 167, 184,

197, 198, 205, 209, 213, 220, 222, 226, 228, 229, 242, 246, 249, 253, 259, 261, 267, 269, 271, 272, 276, 286, 288, 320, 321, 327, 335, 361, 372, 373, 396, 405, 409, 416, 424, 426, 429)

8) Religion

(1, 2, 17, 22, 50, 73, 81, 92, 114, 144, 158, 205, 213, 220, 372, 416, 431)

9) Residential mobility

(1, 2, 22, 32, 184, 205, 206, 210, 228, 229, 314, 363, 372, 401, 403, 419)

2. Enabling

a. Mutable

1) Socioeconomic status and occupation

(1, 2, 13, 17, 19, 23, 24, 27, 32, 35, 37, 47, 50, 52, 56, 62, 64, 69, 71, 73, 74, 84, 89, 92, 104, 108, 110, 114, 115, 117, 121, 124, 130, 133, 140, 141, 142, 145, 153, 158, 162, 174, 181, 184, 193, 196, 201, 202, 205, 210, 211, 213, 215, 216, 221, 222, 228, 229, 267, 272, 307, 308, 310, 313, 320, 321, 324, 327, 328, 332, 335, 337, 342, 344, 351, 353, 355, 361, 363, 375, 387, 390, 391, 397, 399, 402, 403, 404, 405, 414, 415, 416, 417, 418, 424, 425, 429, 430, 431)

2) Income and sources of income

(1, 2, 3, 4, 5, 12, 17, 18, 19, 22, 23, 24, 25, 26, 27, 35, 36, 37, 38, 42, 43, 45, 50, 52, 54, 56, 57, 58, 60, 64, 65, 83, 89, 92, 93, 96, 102, 108, 109, 110, 114, 115, 119, 120, 121, 122, 124, 130, 142, 150, 151, 152, 154, 155, 157, 158, 172, 175, 189, 193, 195, 196, 197, 198, 201, 202, 205, 209, 210, 211, 213, 218, 222, 224, 226, 229, 240, 242, 244, 245, 246, 247, 248, 249, 250, 252, 253, 258, 259, 260, 261, 262, 264, 267, 268, 269, 271, 272, 273, 274, 276, 278, 304, 305, 307, 308, 311, 313, 314, 324, 325, 326, 327, 332, 337, 340, 341, 342, 359, 385, 394, 397, 399, 403, 406, 409, 410, 414, 416, 419, 420, 425, 426, 427, 428, 429)

3) Insurance coverage — type of payer, extent of coverage, method of payment

(1, 2, 3, 4, 5, 12, 15, 17, 18, 19, 20, 22, 24, 27, 36, 37, 38, 40, 41, 43, 47, 52, 54, 60, 62, 64, 65, 74, 79, 83, 85, 87, 88, 92, 96, 102, 109, 110, 113, 119, 123, 130, 138, 142, 145, 148, 150, 152, 153, 157, 162, 166, 172, 175, 186, 188, 189, 195, 203, 205, 209, 211, 213, 218, 220, 240, 249, 263, 267, 272, 291, 299, 307, 310, 311, 312, 315, 317, 318, 319, 320, 325, 335, 337, 341, 342, 346, 347, 352, 361, 372, 373, 375, 376, 381, 382, 385, 394, 395, 397, 399, 403, 404, 406, 409, 412, 416, 419, 423, 426, 427, 428)

4) Price of medical services

(3, 4, 17, 19, 20, 22, 36, 37, 52, 60, 64, 65, 92, 109, 110, 123, 172, 213, 291, 337, 358)

5) Organization of services

(11, 13, 17, 20, 22, 23, 24, 36, 37, 40, 47, 54, 62, 64, 70, 74, 86, 87, 92, 98, 102, 110, 115, 129, 130, 135, 136, 138, 139, 145, 150, 156, 165, 166, 167, 186, 188, 195, 203, 213, 220, 222, 223, 226, 281, 282, 283, 284, 287, 288, 289, 290, 291, 292, 293, 294, 295, 296, 297, 302, 303, 308, 309, 310, 312, 317, 318, 320, 324, 325, 330, 332, 335, 342, 343, 346, 347, 352, 355, 365, 374, 375, 381, 382, 394, 395, 396, 401, 409, 412, 417, 418, 423, 427, 428)

6) Regular source of care

(5, 17, 18, 19, 22, 35, 37, 60, 62, 92, 93, 108, 146, 153, 155, 157, 159, 162, 174, 205, 213, 218, 223, 226, 235, 312, 327, 341, 342, 352, 363, 364, 385, 390, 391, 394, 404, 415)

7) Ease of getting to care

(2, 3, 5, 8, 22, 35, 48, 50, 60, 62, 64, 67, 70, 92, 114, 115, 129, 130, 150, 157, 171, 174, 205, 213, 222, 228, 235, 262, 311, 320, 327, 337, 344, 364, 379, 380, 388, 416, 417, 418, 425, 427)

8) Availability of health resources

(8, 17, 22, 32, 37, 60, 92, 96, 111, 115, 129, 130, 131,
139, 150, 213, 226, 307, 325, 326, 348, 349, 377, 395,
426, 427)

b. Immutable

1) Region
(17, 22, 37, 92, 115, 142, 209, 244, 245, 246, 248, 249,
250, 252, 253, 254, 258, 259, 261, 264, 266, 267, 268,
269, 271, 273, 274, 275, 278, 284, 287, 288, 290, 292,
293, 294, 295, 296, 297, 298, 300, 301, 302, 303, 304,
305, 307, 311, 315, 325, 410, 416)

2) Residence

(1, 2, 8, 17, 18, 19, 21, 22, 23, 24, 26, 27, 32, 36, 38,
42, 43, 47, 65, 92, 104, 108, 109, 115, 142, 151, 209,
244, 245, 248, 249, 250, 252, 253, 254, 258, 261, 264,
267, 268, 269, 271, 273, 274, 275, 278, 281, 299, 304,
305, 307, 311, 312, 323, 324, 325, 326, 339, 361, 380,
385, 391, 400, 406, 415, 416, 425, 427)

3. Need

a. Perceived

1) Health status

(17, 22, 24, 37, 55, 60, 62, 64, 92, 114, 123, 126, 130,
142, 174, 175, 179, 184, 186, 205, 213, 272, 279, 280,
282, 283, 284, 285, 286, 287, 291, 314, 322, 323, 326,
327, 341, 342, 344, 378, 395, 403, 415)

2) Symptoms of illness

(9, 10, 17, 18, 22, 23, 24, 35, 37, 64, 92, 101, 102, 108,
109, 121, 123, 130, 146, 158, 163, 167, 174, 175, 193,
211, 213, 215, 223, 226, 235, 307, 324, 325, 327, 363,
364, 392, 393, 403, 404, 415, 432)

3) Disability days

(5, 17, 21, 22, 24, 26, 37, 60, 62, 65, 92, 121, 142, 157,

163, 171, 175, 205, 213, 223, 224, 235, 240, 241, 242, 243, 255, 257, 263, 265, 267, 268, 270, 272, 273, 275, 277, 279, 280, 282, 283, 284, 285, 286, 287, 291, 311, 314, 325, 326, 327, 342, 406, 416)

4) Chronic activity limitation

(3, 22, 37, 60, 65, 92, 126, 145, 157, 186, 193, 202, 213, 223, 235, 241, 242, 243, 244, 245, 248, 249, 250, 252, 253, 255, 257, 258, 262, 263, 265, 269, 270, 271, 276, 277, 279, 280, 282, 283, 284, 285, 286, 287, 291, 325, 326, 327, 397, 406, 412, 418)

b. Evaluated

1) Medically-defined need

(14, 92, 121, 129, 130, 158, 166, 174, 201, 226, 341, 342, 344, 360, 415, 421)

2) Diagnosis

(15, 22, 35, 37, 40, 41, 47, 86, 92, 98, 113, 115, 117, 121, 124, 126, 129, 130, 137, 139, 144, 145, 146, 165, 174, 189, 202, 203, 213, 220, 223, 228, 235, 241, 242, 243, 244, 252, 255, 257, 263, 265, 269, 270, 271, 273, 275, 277, 279, 280, 282, 283, 284, 285, 286, 287, 288, 291, 292, 293, 294, 295, 296, 297, 301, 304, 305, 325, 327, 340, 342, 358, 363, 364, 388, 392, 393, 418, 428)

3) Surgery

(11, 17, 18, 36, 38, 40, 41, 43, 86, 92, 115, 129, 130, 209, 223, 254, 292, 427)

III.   OUTCOME INDICES

A. *Utilization*

1. Type

a. Hospital

(3, 9, 10, 11, 12, 13, 15, 17, 18, 20, 22, 24, 26, 27, 32, 36, 37, 38, 40, 41, 42, 43, 47, 48, 50, 54, 60, 63, 67, 83, 86,

87, 92, 96, 103, 104, 109, 111, 115, 121, 123, 126, 129,
130, 131, 135, 136, 137, 140, 143, 150, 151, 152, 153,
154, 156, 157, 159, 166, 172, 174, 175, 177, 183, 188,
196, 201, 203, 209, 211, 213, 219, 223, 224, 226, 235,
240, 241, 242, 243, 246, 247, 249, 252, 254, 255, 257,
259, 261, 262, 263, 264, 265, 266, 269, 270, 272, 277,
292, 293, 294, 295, 296, 297, 298, 299, 300, 301, 302,
303, 304, 305, 309, 312, 315, 317, 318, 319, 326, 327,
330, 332, 335, 337, 340, 343, 344, 346, 347, 348, 349,
350, 358, 360, 363, 364, 373, 374, 376, 377, 378, 380,
381, 382, 390, 391, 394, 395, 396, 397, 404, 406, 415,
420, 421, 423, 424, 426, 427, 428)

b. Physician

(1, 2, 3, 4, 5, 9, 10, 11, 12, 13, 14, 17, 18, 19, 20, 21, 22,
23, 24, 26, 27, 29, 35, 36, 37, 38, 40, 42, 43, 47, 50, 51,
52, 54, 55, 56, 57, 58, 60, 62, 63, 64, 65, 67, 69, 70, 71,
73, 74, 77, 78, 79, 81, 83, 84, 85, 89, 92, 93, 98, 100, 101,
102, 104, 108, 109, 113, 114, 117, 120, 121, 123, 126,
133, 135, 136, 138, 140, 141, 142, 143, 144, 145, 146,
150, 151, 152, 153, 154, 156, 157, 158, 163, 167, 170,
171, 172, 175, 177, 179, 184, 186, 189, 193, 194, 195,
196, 202, 209, 210, 211, 213, 215, 216, 218, 221, 222,
223, 224, 226, 228, 229, 235, 242, 243, 244, 245, 247,
249, 252, 254, 257, 258, 261, 262, 263, 264, 265, 269,
270, 272, 273, 277, 304, 305, 310, 311, 312, 318, 320,
321, 322, 323, 324, 325, 326, 327, 332, 335, 337, 340,
341, 342, 342, 346, 350, 351, 352, 353, 355, 356, 357,
359, 361, 372, 373, 374, 375, 378, 380, 381, 382, 384,
385, 386, 387, 388, 392, 393, 394, 395, 396, 397, 399,
400, 401, 403, 405, 406, 408, 409, 410, 414, 416, 418,
419, 420, 424, 425, 426, 427, 428, 429, 430, 431, 432)

c. Dentist

(17, 18, 19, 20, 22, 24, 26, 27, 36, 37, 38, 40, 42, 43, 45,
50, 6o, 69, 71, 73, 74, 92, 93, 100, 122, 150, 153, 172,
177, 180, 181, 182, 196, 197, 198, 210, 242, 243, 247,
248, 249, 250, 254, 261, 263, 264, 265, 269, 270, 274,
277, 304, 307, 308, 313, 327, 328, 334, 340, 361, 365,
373, 380, 397, 399, 405, 406, 419, 420, 426, 427)

d. Nursing and personal care homes

(38, 92, 109, 137, 148, 165, 166, 220, 279, 280, 281, 282, 283, 284, 285, 286, 287, 288, 289, 290, 291, 381)

e. Prescribed and nonprescribed drugs and druggists

(17, 18, 20, 24, 27, 36, 37, 38, 42, 43, 55, 92, 142, 175, 177, 235, 247, 249, 253, 256, 326, 327, 373, 374, 426)

f. Appliances — visual, hearing aids, etc.

(18, 36, 38, 40, 43, 92, 177, 247, 249, 255, 260, 276, 285, 373, 378, 399, 419)

g. Home care

(36, 38, 69, 92, 165, 166, 210, 271, 326, 378, 412)

h. Emergency care or ambulance services

(12, 92, 129, 130, 139, 159, 174, 183, 201, 219, 226, 309, 312, 344, 360, 363, 364, 391, 404, 415, 421)

i. Other — x-rays, lab tests, etc.

(17, 36, 37, 38, 40, 47, 69, 92, 109, 126, 151, 152, 153, 156, 175, 193, 210, 235, 247, 249, 278, 305, 320, 361, 375, 396, 401, 403, 426)

2. Site

(3, 9, 12, 13, 18, 22, 26, 29, 35, 36, 37, 38, 41, 43, 47, 50, 52, 58, 63, 67, 69, 70, 83, 89, 92, 93, 98, 102, 109, 113, 119, 120, 121, 122, 123, 129, 130, 135, 138, 139, 143, 144, 146, 150, 151, 152, 153, 154, 156, 159, 166, 170, 175, 183, 186, 189, 193, 194, 195, 196, 202, 205, 209, 210, 211, 213, 216, 219, 223, 224, 226, 228, 229, 235, 252, 253, 254, 258, 260, 261, 262, 264, 269, 271, 272, 273, 278, 287, 288, 289, 304, 305, 309, 310, 312, 320, 324, 340, 350, 351, 352, 353, 363, 364, 375, 378, 382, 384, 386, 388, 390, 391, 394, 397, 404, 406, 409, 415, 417, 418, 419, 420, 424, 427, 428, 430)

3. Purpose

a. Preventive

(4, 11, 13, 17, 18, 22, 26, 36, 37, 38, 41, 43, 45, 47, 51, 56,
57, 60, 63, 65, 69, 71, 74, 77, 81, 84, 89, 92, 93, 100, 108,
114, 117, 121, 122, 133, 140, 141, 143, 150, 153, 156,
170, 177, 179, 181, 182, 186, 189, 194, 195, 197, 198,
201, 210, 213, 219, 221, 222, 224, 228, 244, 245, 248,
258, 264, 272, 273, 277, 304, 305, 307, 322, 327, 340,
352, 356, 357, 359, 365, 372, 385, 387, 388, 392, 393,
397, 399, 405, 408, 410, 414, 419, 420, 424, 425, 428,
429, 430, 431)

b. Illness-related

(4, 5, 9, 10, 11, 13, 14, 17, 18, 21, 22, 27, 29, 35, 36, 37,
38, 40, 41, 43, 47, 51, 55, 60, 63, 65, 69, 74, 86, 91, 92,
98, 101, 102, 108, 113, 115, 117, 121, 122, 124, 129, 130,
139, 140, 143, 144, 145, 153, 156, 157, 158, 159, 163,
165, 166, 170, 174, 175, 177, 179, 183, 186, 189, 194,
195, 201, 210, 211, 213, 223, 224, 226, 244, 245, 248,
252, 256, 258, 271, 272, 273, 277, 279, 280, 281, 282,
283, 284, 285, 286, 287, 288, 289, 290, 291, 301, 304,
307, 309, 312, 321, 324, 325, 327, 340, 341, 342, 343,
344, 352, 358, 359, 360, 363, 364, 365, 372, 388, 391,
392, 393, 397, 403, 404, 405, 415, 416, 417, 420, 421,
424, 427, 428, 432)

c. Custodial

(22, 36, 38, 63, 92, 137, 165, 166, 220, 271, 279, 280, 281,
282, 283, 284, 285, 286, 287, 288, 289, 290, 291, 412)

4. Time interval

a. Contact

(1, 2, 4, 5, 9, 10, 12, 14, 18, 21, 22, 23, 24, 27, 29, 36, 37,
38, 40, 41, 43, 45, 47, 48, 51, 54, 56, 57, 60, 63, 65, 67,
69, 70, 73, 74, 77, 78, 79, 81, 84, 85, 86, 91, 92, 93, 98,
100, 101, 103, 104, 108, 113, 120, 121, 122, 123, 129,
130, 133, 135, 138, 140, 141, 143, 144, 145, 151, 152,

153, 154, 156, 157, 158, 163, 165, 170, 174, 177, 180,
181, 182, 183, 184, 189, 193, 196, 197, 198, 201, 205,
206, 209, 210, 211, 213, 219, 220, 223, 225, 226, 228,
229, 235, 242, 243, 244, 245, 246, 247, 250, 252, 255,
256, 258, 259, 260, 261, 264, 269, 270, 271, 273, 274,
276, 277, 278, 279, 280, 281, 282, 283, 284, 285, 286,
287, 288, 289, 290, 291, 300, 301, 303, 304, 305, 307,
308, 309, 310, 312, 322, 324, 325, 326, 327, 335, 337,
340, 341, 342, 344, 351, 352, 359, 360, 363, 364, 365,
372, 378, 380, 387, 391, 392, 393, 397, 399, 403, 408,
409, 410, 412, 414, 415, 417, 419, 420, 421, 424, 425,
427, 428, 429, 430, 431, 432)

b. Volume

(3, 4, 5, 9, 10, 11, 13, 15, 17, 18, 19, 20, 21, 22, 24, 26, 27,
29, 32, 35, 36, 37, 38, 40, 41, 42, 43, 45, 47, 55, 60, 62,
63, 64, 65, 69, 70, 81, 83, 86, 87, 88, 91, 92, 96, 102, 104,
108, 110, 111, 113, 115, 117, 120, 121, 123, 126, 129,
130, 131, 135, 136, 139, 142, 143, 145, 148, 150, 151,
152, 153, 154, 156, 157, 159, 166, 170, 171, 172, 173,
175, 177, 186, 188, 195, 196, 202, 203, 206, 209, 210,
213, 218, 220, 221, 222, 223, 224, 226, 228, 229, 235,
240, 241, 242, 243, 244, 245, 246, 247, 248, 249, 252,
253, 254, 255, 256, 257, 258, 259, 261, 262, 263, 264,
265, 266, 269, 270, 272, 273, 274, 276, 277, 278, 279,
280, 281, 282, 283, 284, 285, 286, 287, 288, 289, 290,
291, 292, 293, 294, 295, 296, 297, 298, 299, 300, 301,
302, 303, 304, 305, 307, 308, 309, 310, 311, 313, 315,
317, 318, 319, 320, 321, 322, 323, 324, 325, 326, 327,
328, 330, 332, 335, 337, 340, 341, 342, 343, 346, 347,
348, 349, 351, 352, 353, 355, 359, 361, 365, 373, 374,
375, 376, 377, 378, 381, 382, 385, 388, 391, 392, 393,
394, 395, 396, 397, 401, 404, 405, 406, 409, 416, 417,
418, 420, 423, 424, 426, 427, 428)

c. Continuity

(13, 14, 22, 35, 37, 52, 55, 56, 63, 67, 70, 73, 74, 91, 92,
113, 114, 121, 124, 130, 137, 143, 145, 146, 147, 151,
152, 154, 159, 165, 166, 167, 170, 175, 213, 215, 216,
219, 223, 226, 228, 229, 246, 259, 307, 310, 312, 324,
341, 342, 363, 364, 374, 384, 385, 386, 390, 391, 392,
393, 394, 400, 404, 412, 428)

5. Bibliographic references on utilization

(6, 92, 130, 208, 217, 227, 413)

B. *Consumer Satisfaction*

(8, 13, 25, 44, 48, 55, 70, 97, 101, 102, 108, 121, 153, 159, 161, 162, 207, 225, 312, 314, 339, 350, 394)

IV. RELATED METHODOLOGICAL ISSUES

A. *Measurement — Index Construction*

1. Social indicators — general

(34, 44, 53, 72, 80, 95, 116, 118, 128, 200, 354, 383, 389, 398, 407)

2. Social indicators — health status

(34, 46, 61, 99, 107, 132, 134, 168, 169, 187, 212, 231, 233, 236, 306, 316, 329, 362)

3. Bibliographic references on social indicators

(7, 190, 191, 192, 230, 422)

B. *Evaluation — Quality of Care*

(49, 68, 75, 106, 127, 160, 164, 176, 331, 338, 366, 367, 368, 369, 370)

C. *Data Collection*

(214, 232, 234, 237, 238, 239, 336)

D. *Data Analysis*

(28, 30, 31, 33, 34, 94, 199, 333, 345)

Bibliography

1. Abernathy, W.J. and J.R. Moore
   1972   "Regional planning of primary health care ser-
           vices." *Med. Care* 10 (September-October):
           380-394.

2. Abernathy, W.J. and E.L. Schrems
   1971   "Distance and health services: issues of utilization
           and facility choice for demographic strata." Re-
           search Paper No. 19. Palo Alto: Graduate School of
           Business, Stanford University.

3. Acton, J.P.
   1972   "Demand for health care among the urban poor,
           with special emphasis on the role of time." Unpub.
           manuscript. Santa Monica, California: Rand Corpo-
           ration.

4. Aday, L.A.
   1971   "Dimensions of family's social status and their rela-
           tionships to children's utilization of health ser-
           vices." Unpublished manuscript. Baltimore: De-
           partment of Medical Care and Hospitals, Johns
           Hopkins University.

5. Aday, L.A.
   1973   "Economic and non-economic barriers to the use of
           needed medical services." Unpub. Ph.D. disserta-
           tion. Lafayette, Indiana: Department of Sociology,
           Purdue University.

6. Aday, L.A. and R.L. Eichhorn
   1972   *The Utilization of Health Services: Indices and Cor-
           relates. A Research Bibliography.* Washington: Na-
           tional Center for Health Services Research and De-
           velopment: U.S. Dept. HEW Publication No.
           (HSM) 73-3003.

7. Agency for International Development
   1972   *Social Indicators: A Selected List of References for
           AID Technicians.* Washington: AID Bibliography
           Series: Technical Assistance Methodology No. 2.

8. Albrecht, S.L. and M.K. Miller
   1973   "Health service delivery: an assessment of some adequacy indicators." Paper presented at the Rural Sociology Society meetings, Baltimore (August).

9. Alpert, J.J., et al.
   1967a   "A month of illness and health care among low-income families." *Public Health Rep.* 82 (August): 705-713.

10. Alpert, J.J., et al.
    1967b   "Medical help and maternal nursing care in the life of low-income families." *Pediatrics* 39 (May): 749-755.

11. Alpert, J.J., et al.
    1968   "Effective use of comprehensive pediatric care." *Amer. J. Dis. Child* 116 (November): 529-533.

12. Alpert, J.J., et al.
    1969   "Types of families that use an emergency clinic." *Med. Care* 7 (January-February): 55-61.

13. Alpert, J.J., et al.
    1970   "Attitudes and satisfaction of low-income families receiving comprehensive pediatric care." *Amer. J. Public Health* 60 (March): 499-506.

14. Ambuel, J.P., et al.
    1964   "Urgency as a factor in clinic attendance." *Amer. J. Dis. Child* 4 (October): 394-398.

15. Ament, R.P.
    1967   "Medicare boosts bed usage by elderly." *Mod. Hosp.* 108 (February): 81-82.

16. American Medical Association
    1973   *Contributions to a Comprehensive Health Manpower Strategy.* AMA: Center for Health Services Research and Development.

17. Andersen, R.
    1968   *A Behavioral Model of Families' Use of Health Services.* Research Series No. 25. Chicago: Center for Health Administration Studies, University of Chicago

18. Andersen, R. and O.W. Anderson
   1967   *A Decade of Health Services.* Chicago: University
             of Chicago Press.

19. Andersen, R. and L. Benham
   1970   "Factors affecting the relationship between family
             income and medical care consumption." In H.E.
             Klarman (ed.), *Empirical Studies in Health
             Economics.* Baltimore: The Johns Hopkins Press.

20. Andersen, R. and J.T. Hull
   1969   "Hospital utilization and cost trends in Canada and
             the United States." *Med. Care* 7 (November-
             December): 4-22.

21. Andersen, R. and J. Kravits
   1971   "Disability days and physician contact for the two
             week period preceding the interview date by age,
             sex, race, residence, and family income." Prelimi-
             nary Report No. 1 of research conducted under Con-
             tract Number HSM 110-70-392, NCHSRD. Chi-
             cago: Center for Health Administration Studies,
             University of Chicago.

22. Andersen, R. and J. Newman
   1973   "Societal and individual determinants of medical
             care utilization." *Milb. Mem. Fund Quart.* 51
             (Winter): 95-124.

23. Andersen, R., et al.
   1968   "Perceptions of and response to symptoms of illness
             in Sweden and the United States." *Med. Care* 6
             (January-February): 18-30.

24. Andersen, R., et al.
   1970   *Medical Care Use in Sweden and the United States:
             A Comparative Analysis of Systems and Behavior.*
             Research Series No. 27. Chicago: Center for Health
             Administration Studies, University of Chicago.

25. Andersen, R., et al.
   1971   "The public's view of the crisis in medical care: an
             impetus for changing delivery systems?" *Econ. &
             Bus. Bulletin* 24 (Fall): 44-52.

26. Andersen, R., et al.
   1972   *Health Service Use: National Trends and Varia-*

tions — 1953-1971. Washington: National Center for Health Services Research and Development: U.S. Dept. HEW Publication No. (HSM) 73-3004.

27. Andersen, R., et al.
    1973   *Expenditures for Personal Health Services: National Trends and Variations — 1953-1970.* Washington: Bureau of Health Services Research and Evaluation: U.S. Dept. HEW Publication No. (HRA) 74-3105.

28. Anderson, J.G.
    1971a   "Path analysis: A new approach to modeling health service delivery systems." Paper presented at the Joint National Conference on Major Systems, National Meeting of the Operations Research Society of America, Anaheim, California (October 27-29).

29. Anderson, J.G.
    1971b   "Sociocultural variations in response to illness: a comparative study of Anglo-Americans and Spanish Americans." Unpub. manuscript. Lafayette, Indiana: Department of Sociology, Purdue University.

30. Anderson, J.G.
    1972a   "A structural equation model of a health care system." Working Paper No. 52. Lafayette, Indiana: Institute for the Study of Social Change, Department of Sociology, Purdue University.

31. Anderson, J.G.
    1972b   "Causal model of a health services system." *Health Services Research* 7 (Spring):23-42.

32. Anderson, J.G.
    1972c   "Demographic factors affecting health services utilization: a causal model." *Med. Care* 11 (March-April): 104-120.

33. Anderson, J.G.
    1972d   "Social indicators and second-order consequences of health care delivery." *AIIE Transactions* 5 (March): 49-59.

34. Anderson, J.G.
    1973   "Causal models and social indicators: toward the

development of social systems models." *ASR* 38 (June): 285-301.

35. Anderson, J.G. and D.E. Bartkus
    1972   "Choice of medical care: a behavioral model of health and illness behavior." Working Paper No. 63. Lafayette, Indiana: Institute for the Study of Social Change, Department of Sociology, Purdue University.

36. Anderson, O.W.
    1963   "The utilization of health services." In Freeman, H.E., et al. (eds.), *Handbook of Medical Sociology*. Englewood Cliffs: Prentice-Hall.

37. Anderson, O.W.
    1972   *Health Care: Can There Be Equity?* New York: John Wiley and Sons.

38. Anderson, O.W. and R. Andersen
    1972   "Patterns of use of health services." In Freeman, H.E., et al. (eds.), *Handbook of Medical Sociology*. Englewood Cliffs: Prentice-Hall.

39. Anderson, O.W. and J.J. Feldman
    1956   *Family Medical Costs and Voluntary Health Insurance: A Nationwide Survey*. New York: McGraw-Hill Book Co., Inc.

40. Anderson, O.W. and P.B. Sheatsley
    1959   *Comprehensive Medical Insurance: A Study of Costs, Use and Attitudes under Two Plans*. Research Series No. 9. Chicago: Center for Health Administration Studies, University of Chicago.

41. Anderson, O.W. and P.B. Sheatsley
    1967   *Hospital Use — A Survey of Patient and Physician Decisions*. Research Series No. 24. Chicago: Center for Health Administration Studies, University of Chicago.

42. Anderson, O.W., et al.
    1960   *Family Expenditure Patterns for Personal Health Services — 1953 and 1958: Nationwide Surveys*. Research Series No. 14. Chicago: Center for Health Administration Studies, University of Chicago.

43. Anderson, O.W., et al.
    1963   *Changes in Family Medical Care Expenditures and Voluntary Health Insurance.* Cambridge: Harvard University Press.

44. Andrews, F.M. and S.B. Withey
    1973   "Developing measures of perceived life quality: results from several national surveys." Paper presented at the annual meeting of the American Sociological Association, New York City (August).

45. Antonovsky, A. and R. Kats
    1970   "The model dental patient: an empirical study of preventive health behavior." *Soc. Sci. Med.* 4 (November): 367-380.

46. Austin, C.J.
    1971   "Selected social indicators in the health field." *Amer. J. Public Health* 61 (August): 1507-1513.

47. Avnet, H.H.
    1967   *Physician Service Patterns and Illness Rates.* New York: Group Health Insurance, Inc.

48. Baggish, D.A. and C.P. Kimball
    1973   "The problem of transportation to medical facilities on an Indian reservation." *Med. Care* 11 (November-December): 501-508.

49. Banks, F.R. and M.D. Keller
    1971   "Symptoms experienced and health action." *Med. Care* 9 (November-December): 498-502.

50. Bashshur, R.L., et al.
    1971   "Some ecological differentials in the use of medical services." *Health Services Research* 6 (Spring): 61-75.

51. Battistella, R.M.
    1968   "Limitations in the use of the concept of psychological readiness to initiate health care." *Med. Care* 6 (July-August): 308-319.

52. Battistella, R.M.
    1971   "Factors associated with delay in the initiation of physicians' care among late adulthood persons." *Amer. J. Public Health* 61 (July): 1348-1361.

53. Bauer, R.A.
    1966   *Social Indicators.* Cambridge: MIT Press.

54. Beck, R.G.
    1973   "Economic class and access to physician services under public medical care insurance." *Intl. J. Health Services* 3 (Summer): 341-355.

55. Becker, M.H., et al.
    1972   "Motivations as predictors of health behavior." *Health Services Reports* 87 (November): 852-862.

56. Bellin, S.S. and H.J. Geiger
    1972   "The impact of a neighborhood health center on patients' behavior and attitudes relating to health care: a study of a low income housing project." *Med. Care* 10 (May-June): 224-239.

57. Bergner, L. and A. Yerby
    1968   "Low income and barriers to use of health services." *New Eng. J. Med.* 278 (March 7): 541-546.

58. Berkanovic, E. and L.G. Reeder
    1973   "Ethnic, economic and social psychological factors in the source of medical care." *Social Problems* 20 (Fall): 246-259.

59. Bible, B.L.
    1970   "Physician's views of medical practice in non-metropolitan communities." *Public Health Rep.* 85 (January): 11-17.

60. Bice, T.W.
    1971   "Medical care for the disadvantaged: report on a survey of use of medical services in the Baltimore Standard Metropolitan Statistical Area 1968-1969." Final report of research conducted under Contract Number HSM 110-69-203, NCHSRD.

61. Bice, T.W.
    1973   "Comments on health indicators: methodological perspectives." Paper presented at the Seminar on Health Indicators, Columbia University, New York.

62. Bice, T.W. and K.L. White
    1969   "Factors related to the use of health services: an

international comparative study." *Med. Care* 8
(March-April): 124-133.

63. Bice, T.W. and K.L. White
    1971   "Cross-national comparative research on the utiliza-
                tion of medical services." *Med. Care* 9 (May-June):
                253-271.

64. Bice, T.W., et al.
    1972   "Socioeconomic status and use of physicians' ser-
                vices: a reconsideration." *Med. Care* 12 (May-
                June): 261-271.

65. Bice, T.W., et al.
    1973   "Economic class and use of physician services."
                Med. Care 11 (July-August): 287-296.

66. Bodenheimer, T.S.
    1970   "Patterns of American ambulatory care." *Inquiry* 8
                (September): 26-35.

67. Borkow, G.
    1973   "Use of alternate facilities by consumers at the Pro-
                vidence Health Centers." *Inquiry* 10 (March):
                54-58.

67. Brenner, M.H. and H. Paris
    1973   "Record systems for hospital outpatient clinics."
                Med. Care 11 (March-April Supplement): 41-50.

69. Brightman, I., et al.
    1958   "Knowledge and utilization of health resources by
                public assistance recipients." *Amer. J. Public
                Health* 48 (February): 188-199.

70. Brooks, C.H.
    1973   "Associations among distance, patient satisfaction,
                and utilization of two types of inner-city clinics."
                Med. Care 11 (September-October): 373-383.

71. Bullough, B.
    1972   "Poverty, ethnic identity and preventive health
                care." *J. Health Soc. Behav.* 13 (December):
                347-359.

72. Campbell, A. and P. Converse
    1970   "Monitoring the quality of American life." A proposal to the Russell Sage Foundation. Ann Arbor, Michigan: Survey Research Center, University of Michigan.

73. Cauffman, J.G., et al.
    1967c   "Medical care of school children: factors influencing outcome of referral from a school health program." *Amer. J. Public Health* 57 (January): 60-73.

74. Cauffman, J.G., et al.
    1967b   "The impact of health insurance coverage on health care of school children." *Public Health Rep.* 82 (April): 323-328.

75. Center for Health Administration Studies
    1973   *The Hospital's Role in Assessing the Quality of Medical Care: Proceedings of the Fifteenth Annual Symposium on Hospital Affairs.* Chicago: Center for Health Administration Studies, University of Chicago.

76. Chen, M.K.
    1973   "Access to health care: a preliminary model." Unpub. manuscript. National Center for Health Services Research and Development.

77. Clausen, J.A., et al.
    1954   "Parent attitudes toward participation of their children in polio vaccine trials." *Amer. J. Public Health* 44 (December): 1526-1536.

78. Coe, R.M. and A. Wessen
    1965   "Social psychological factors influencing the use of community health resources." *Amer. J. Public Health* 55 (July) 1024-1031.

79. Coe, R.M., et al.
    1967   "The impact of Medicare on the utilization and provision of health care facilities: a sociological interpretation." *Inquiry* 4 (December): 42-46.

80. Coleman, J.S.
    1971   "Problems of conceptualization and measurement in studying policy impacts." Paper presented at the Conference on the Impact of Public Policies, St. Thomas, U.S. Virgin Islands (December 3-5).

81. Collver, A., et al.
    1967   "Factors influencing the use of maternal health services." *Soc. Sci. Med.* 1 (September): 293-308.

82. Crawford, C.O.
    1971   "Some relevant concerns and issues in research on personal health delivery systems with special emphasis on nonmetropolitan areas." In *Working Papers on Rural Community Services* compiled by S.M. Leadly, Department of Agricultural Economic and Rural Sociology, The Pennsylvania State University for the National Workshop on Problems of Research on Delivery of Community Services in Rural Areas, Lincoln, Nebraska (December 13-16).

83. Darsky, B.J., et al.
    1958   *Comprehensive Medical Services Under Voluntary Health Insurance: A Study of Windsor Medical Services.* Cambridge: Harvard University Press.

84. Deasy, L.
    1956   "Socioeconomic status and participation in the poliomyelitis vaccine trial." *ASR* 21 (April): 185-191.

85. Densen, P.M., et al.
    1959   "Concerning high and low utilizers of services on a medical care plan, and the persistence of utilization levels over a three-year period." *Milb. Mem. Fund Quart.* 37 (July): 217-250.

86. Densen, P.M., et al.
    1960   "Prepaid medical care and hospital utilization in a dual choice situation." *Amer. J. Public Health* 50 (November): 1710-1726.

87. Densen, P.M., et al.
    1962   "Prepaid medical care and hospital utilization: comparison of a group practice and self-insurance situation." *Hospitals* 36 (November 16): 63-68; 138.

88. Diokno, A.W.
    1962   "Relationship between benefit levels and hospital utilization." In McNerny, W.J., et al., *Hospital and Medical Economics.* Chicago: Hospital Research and Educational Trust.

89. Dodge, W.F., et al.
    1970   "Patterns of maternal desires for child health care."
            Amer. J. Public Health 60 (August): 1421-1429.

90. Donabedian, A.
    1969   "An evaluation of prepaid group practice." *Inquiry*
            6 (September): A-1—A-25.

91. Donabedian, A.
    1972   "Models for organizing the delivery of personal
            health services and criteria for evaluating them."
            Milb. Mem. Fund Quart. 50 (October): 103-154.

92. Donabedian, A.
    1973   *Aspects of Medical Care Administration.*
            Cambridge: Harvard University Press.

93. Donabedian, A. and L.S. Rosenfeld
    1961   "Some factors influencing prenatal care." *New
            Eng. J. Med.* 265 (July 6): 1-6.

94. Duncan, O.D.
    1966   "Path analysis: sociological examples." *AJS* 72
            (July): 1-17.

95. Duncan, O.D.
    1969   *Toward Social Reporting: Next Steps.* New York:
            Russell Sage Foundation.

96. Durbin, R.L. and G. Antelman
    1964   "A study of the effects of selected variables on hos-
            pital utilization." *Hospital Manage.* 98 (August):
            57-60.

97. Edwards, A.L.
    1957   *Techniques of Attitude Scale Construction.* New
            York: Appleton-Century-Crofts, Inc.

98. Elford, R.W., et al.
    1972   "A study of house calls in the practices of general
            practitioners." *Med. Care* 10 (September-October):
            380-394.

99. Elinson, J., et al.
    1973   "Toward sociomedical health indicators." Paper
            presented at International Conference of Medical
            Sociology, Warsaw, Poland (August 20-25).

100. Ellenbogen, B.L., et al.
     1968   "The diffusion of two preventive health practices."
               Inquiry 5 (June): 62-71.

101. Elliott, J.L.
     1972   "Cultural barriers to the utilization of health ser-
               vices." *Inquiry* 9 (December): 28-35.

102. Enterline, P., et al.
     1973   "The distribution of medical services before and
               after 'free' medical care — the Quebec experience."
               New Eng. J. Med. 289 (November 29): 1174-1178.

103. Fabrega, H., Jr. and R.E. Roberts
     1972a   "Ethnic differences in the outpatient use of a
               public-charity hospital." *Amer. J. Public Health* 62
               (July): 936-941.

104. Fabrega, H., Jr. and R.E. Roberts
     1972b   "Social psychological correlates of physician use by
               economically disadvantaged Negro urban resi-
               dents." *Med. Care* 10 (May-June): 215-223.

105. Falk, I.S.
     1933   *The Incidence of Illness and Receipt and Costs of
               Medical Care among Representative Families: Ex-
               periences in 12 Consecutive Months During
               1928-1931.* Chicago: University of Chicago Press.

106. Falk, I.S., et al.
     1967   "The development of standards for the audit and
               planning of medical care. I. Concepts, research de-
               sign, and the content of primary physicians' care."
               Amer. J. Public Health 57 (July): 1118-1136.

107. Fanshel, S. and J.W. Bush
     1970   "A health-status index and its application to health-
               services outcomes." *Operations Research* 18
               (November-December): 1021-1066.

108. Feldman, J.J.
     1966   *The Dissemination of Health Information.* Chicago:
               Aldine Publishing Company.

109. Feldstein, P.J.
     1966   "Research on the demand for health services."
               Milb. Mem. Fund Quart. 44 (July): 128-162.

110. Feldstein, P.J. and J.W. Carr
   1964   "The effect of income on medical care spending."
             Proceedings of the Social Statistics Section, Ameri-
             can Statistical Association: 93-105.

111. Feldstein, P.J. and J.J. German
   1965   "Predicting hospital utilization: an evaluation of
             three approaches." *Inquiry* 2 (June): 13-36.

112. Fenderson, D.A.
   1973   "Health manpower development and rural ser-
             vices." *JAMA* (September 24): 1627-1631.

113. Fink, R.
   1973   "Analysis of utilization data." *Med. Care* 11
             (March-April Supplement): 109-116.

114. Fink, R., et al.
   1968   "The reluctant participant in breast cancer screen-
             ing programs." *Public Health Rep.* 83 (June):
             479-490.

115. Fitzpatrick, T.B., et al.
   1962   "Character and effectiveness of hospital use." In
             McNerny, W.J., et al., *Hospital and Medical
             Economics.* Chicago: Hospital Research and Edu-
             cational Trust.

116. Flax, M.J.
   1971   "Future prospects for the development of additional
             social and urban indicators." Working Paper No.
             1206-2. Washington: The Urban Institute.

117. Foster, A., et al.
   1973   "Use of health services in relation to the physical
             home environment of an Indian population." *Public
             Health Rep.* 88 (October): 715-720.

118. Fox, K.A.
   1971   "Combining economic and noneconomic objectives
             in development planning: problems of concept and
             measurement." Unpub. manuscript. Ames, Iowa:
             Department of Economics, Iowa State University.

119. Fox, P.D.
   1972   "Access to medical care for the poor: the federal
             perspective." *Med. Care* 10 (May-June): 272-277.

120. Franklin, B.J. and S.D. McLemore
     1970   "Factors affecting the choice of medical care among
               university students." *J. Health Soc. Behav.* 11 (De-
               cember): 311-319.

121. Freeborn, D.K. and M.R. Greenlick
     1973   "Evaluation of the performance of ambulatory care
               systems: research equipments and opportunities."
               Med. Care 11 (March-April Supplement): 68-75.

122. Freeman, H.E. and C. Lambert, Jr.
     1965   "Preventive dental behavior of urban mothers." *J.
               Health Hum. Behav.* 6 (Fall): 141-147.

123. Freeman, H.E., et al.
     1966   "Use of medical resources by SPANCOS: I. extent
               and sources of medical care in a very old popula-
               tion." *Amer. J. Public Health* 56 (September):
               1530-1539.

124. Friedman, B., et al.
     1973   "The influence of medical and private health insur-
               ance on the early diagnosis of breast cancer." *Med.
               Care* 11 (November-December): 485-490.

125. Freidson, E. and J.H. Mann
     1971   "Organizational dimensions of large-scale group
               practice." *Amer. J. Public Health* 61 (April):
               786-795.

126. Gaspard, N.J. and E.E. Hopkins
     1967   "Determinants of use of ambulatory medical ser-
               vices by an aged population." *Inquiry* 4 (March):
               28-36.

127. Gavett, J.W., et al.
     1973   "Physician judgments and resource utilization in a
               private practice." *Med. Care* 11 (July-August):
               310-319.

128. Gessaman, P.H. and G.D. Rose
     1971   "Problems of measurement and assessment of the
               adequacy of community services: A naive view-
               point." In *Working Papers on Rural Community
               Services* compiled by S.M. Leadley, Department of
               Agricultural Economics and Rural Sociology, The

Pennsylvania State University for the National Workshop on Problems of Research on Delivery of Community Services in Rural Areas Lincoln, Nebraska (December 13-16).

129. Gibson, G.
1973 "Evaluative criteria for emergency ambulance systems." *Soc. Sci. Med.* 7 (June): 425-454.

130. Gibson, G., et al.
1970 *Emergency Medical Services in the Chicago Area.* Chicago: Center for Health Administration Studies, University of Chicago.

131. Gish, O.
1973 "Resource allocation, equality of access, and health." *Intl. J. Health Services* 3 (Summer): 399-412.

132. Gitter, A.G. and D.I. Mostofsky
1972 "Toward a social indicator of health." *Soc. Sci. Med.* 6 (April): 205-209.

133. Glasser, M.A.
1958 "Study of the public's acceptance of the Salk vaccine program." *Amer. J. Public Health* 48 (February): 141-146.

134. Goldsmith, S.B.
1972 "The status of health status indicators." *Health Services Reports* 87 (March): 212-220.

135. Goodrich, C.H., et al.
1965 "A progress report on an experiment in welfare medical care." *Amer. J. Public Health* 55 (January): 88-93.

136. Goodrich, C.H., et al.
1970 *Welfare Medical Care.* Cambridge: Harvard University Press.

137. Gordon, D.W.
1973 "Post-hospital discharge: patient care and utilization of services and facilities." *Inquiry* 10 (December): 41-48.

138. Gornick, M.E., et al.
     1969   "Use of medical services as demanded by the urban
               poor." *Amer. J. Public Health* 59 (August):
               1302-1311.

139. Graf, W.S., et al.
     1973   "A community program for emergency cardiac care:
               a three-year coronary ambulance paramedic evalua-
               tion." *JAMA* 226 (October 8): 150-160.

140. Graham, S.
     1957   "Socioeconomic status, illness and use of medical
               services." *Milb. Mem. Fund Quart.* 36 (January):
               58-66.

141. Gray, R.M., et al.
     1966   "The effects of social class and friends' expectations
               on oral polio vaccination participation." *Amer. J.
               Public Health* 56 (December): 2028-2032.

142. Green, J. and J. Scharff
     1971   "Use of medical services under Medicare." *Soc.
               Sec. Bull.* 34 (March): 3-16.

143. Greenlick, M.R. and D.K. Freeborn
     1971   "Determinants of medical care utilization: on choos-
               ing the appropriate measure of utilization." Paper
               presented at the Engineering Foundation Confer-
               ence on Qualitative Decision Making for the Deliv-
               ery of Ambulatory Care, Henniker, New Hamp-
               shire (July).

144. Greenlick, M.R., et al.
     1968   "Determinants of medical care utilization." *Health
               Services Research* 3 (Winter): 296-315.

145. Greenlick, M.R., et al.
     1972   "Comparing the use of medical care services by a
               medically indigent and a general membership popu-
               lation and a comprehensive prepaid group practice
               program." *Med. Care* 10 (May-June): 187-200.

146. Greenlick, M.R., et al.
     1973   "Determinants of medical care utilization: the role
               of the telephone in total medical care." *Med. Care* 11
               (March-April): 121-134.

147. Hackett, T.P., et al.
1973   "Patient delay in cancer." *New Eng. J. Med.* 289 (July 5): 14-20.

148. Harmon, E.L.
1968   "Third-party payment increases utilization of home care services." *Hospitals* 42 (September 1): 68-72.

149. Hassinger, E.W.
1963   *Background and Community Orientation of Rural Physicians Compared with Metropolitan Physicians in Missouri.* Research Bulletin 822. Columbia, Missouri: Agricultural Experiment Station, College of Agriculture, University of Missouri.

150. Hassinger, E.W. and J.C. Belcher
1973   "Patterns of access to health services in rural areas." Unpub. manuscript. Columbia, Missouri: Department of Rural Sociology, University of Missouri.

151. Hassinger, E.W. and D.J. Hobbs
1972   *Health Service Patterns in Rural and Urban Areas: A Test Between Availability and Use.* Research Bulletin 987. Columbia, Missouri: Agricultural Experiment Station, College of Agriculture, University of Missouri.

152. Hassinger, E.W. and D. Hobbs
1973   "The relation of community context to utilization of health services in a rural area." *Med. Care* 11 (November-December): 509-522.

153. Hassinger, E.W. and R.L. McNamara
1973   *Changes in Health Behavior and Opinions Among Open-Country Families in Two Missouri Counties 1955-56 and 1968.* Research Bulletin 994. Columbia, Missouri: Agricultural Experiment Station, College of Agriculture, University of Missouri.

154. Hassinger, E.W., et al.
1970   *Extent, Type and Pattern of Use of Medical Services in a Rural Ozark Area.* Research Bulletin 965. Columbia, Missouri: Agricultural Experiment Station, College of Agriculture, University of Missouri.

155. Hassinger, E.W., et al.
     1971   *Perception of Health Practitioners by Respondents
                 in a Rural Area.* Research Bulletin 964. Columbia
                 Missouri: Agricultural Experiment Station, College
                 of Agriculture, University of Missouri.

156. Hastings, J.E.F., et al.
     1973   "Prepaid group practice in Sault Ste. Marie, On-
                 tario. Part 1. Analysis of utilization records." *Med.
                 Care* 11 (March-April): 91-103.

157. Health Services Research and Training Program
     1972   *Health Services Data System: The Family Health
                 Survey.* Lafayette, Indiana: Health Services Re-
                 search and Training Program, Purdue University.

158. Hetherington, R.W. and C.E. Hopkins
     1969   "Symptom sensitivity: its social and cultural corre-
                 lates." *Health Services Research* 4 (Spring): 63-75.

159. Hillman, B. and E. Charney
     1972   "A neighborhood health center: what the patients
                 know and think of its operation." *Med. Care* 10
                 (July-August): 336-344.

160. Hulka, B.S. and J.C. Cassell
     1973   "The AAFP-UNC study of the organization, utili-
                 zation, and assessment of primary medical care."
                 Amer. J. Public Health 63 (June): 494-501.

161. Hulka, B.S., et al.
     1970   "Scale for the measurement of attitudes toward
                 physicians and primary care." *Med. Care* 8
                 (September-October): 429-436.

162. Hulka, B.S., et al.
     1971   "Satisfaction with medical care in a low-income
                 population." *J. Chronic Dis.* 24 (November):
                 661-673.

163. Hulka, B.S., et al.
     1972   "Determinants of physician utilization: approach to
                 a service-oriented classification of symptoms. *Med.
                 Care* 10 (July-August): 300-309.

164. Hurtado, A.V. and M.R. Greenlick
     1971   "A disease classification system for the analysis of

medical care utilization." *Health Services Research* 6 (Summer): 235-250.

165. Hurtado, A.V., et al.
1969   "The organization and utilization of home-care and extended-care facility as a pre-paid comprehensive group practice plan." *Med. Care* 7 (January-February): 30-40.

166. Hurtado, A.V., et al.
1972   "The utilization and cost of home care and extended care facility services in a comprehensive prepaid group practice program." *Med. Care* 10 (January-February): 8-16.

167. Hurtado, A.V., et al.
1973   "Determinants of medical care utilization: failure to keep appointments." *Med. Care* 11 (May-June): 189-198.

168. Institute for Interdisciplinary Studies
1970   *Social Indicators for the Aged.* Minneapolis, Minnesota: Quantitative Social Planning Division, Institute for Interdisciplinary Studies, American Rehabilitation Foundation.

169. Iowa State Department of Health, Records and Statistics Division
1970   *Measures of Health Status for Counties and Regions in Iowa 1965-1969.* Des Moines, Iowa: Office of Comprehensive Health Planning.

170. Jacobs, A.R. and J.W. Gavett
1973   "Case classification of ambulatory care demand." *Amer. J. Public Health* 63 (August): 721-726.

171. Jehlik, P.J. and R.L. McNamara
1952   "The relation of distance to the differential use of certain health personnel and facilities and the extent of bad illness." *Rural Sociology* 17 (September): 261-265.

172. Joseph, H.
1971   "Empirical research on the demand for health care." *Inquiry* 86 (March): 61-72.

173. Josephson, C.
1966   "Family expenditure patterns of federal employees

for covered items of health care services." *Inquiry* 3 (February): 40-54.

174. Kahn, L., et al.
     1973   "Patient's perceptions and uses of a pediatric emergency room." *Soc. Sci. Med.* 7 (February): 155-160.

175. Kaitaranta, H. and T. Purola
     1973   "A systems-oriented approach to the consumption of medical commodities." *Soc. Sci. Med.* 7 (July): 531-540.

176. Kalimo, E. and K. Sievers
     1968   "The need for medical care: estimation on the basis of interview data." *Med. Care* 6 (January-February): 1-17.

177. Kalimo, E., et al.
     1972   "Interrelationships in the use of selected health services: a cross-national study." *Med. Care* 10 (March-April): 95-108.

178. Kaplan, R.S. and S. Leinhardt
     1973   "Determinants of physician office location." *Med. Care* 11 (September-October): 406-415.

179. Kasl, S. and S. Cobb
     1966   "Health behavior, illness behavior and sick-role behavior." *Arch. Environ. Health* 12 (February): 245-266.

180. Kegeles, S.S.
     1961a   "Why people seek dental care: a review of present knowledge." *Amer. J. Public Health* 51 (September): 1306-1311.

181. Kegeles, S.S.
     1961b   "Why people seek dental care: a test of conceptual formulation. *J. Health Hum. Behav.* 4 (Fall): 166-173.

182. Kegeles, S.S.
     1963   "Some motives for seeking preventive dental care." *J. Amer. Dent. Assoc.* 67 (July): 91-98.

183. Keller, G.B. and M.D. Keller
    1973   "Concepts of sensitivity and specificity in the evaluation of emergency medical services." *Soc. Sci. Med.* 7 (November) 861-864.

184. Kessel, N. and M. Shepard
    1965   "The health and attitudes of people who seldom consult a doctor." *Med. Care* 3 (January-March): 6-10.

185. Kimbell, L.J. and J.H. Lorant
    1973   "Methods for systematic and efficient classification of medical practices." *Health Services Research* 8 (Spring): 46-60.

186. Kisch, A.I. and J.W. Kovner
    1969   "The relationship between health status and utilization of outpatient health services." *Arch. Environ. Health* 18 (May): 820-833.

187. Kisch, A.I., et al.
    1968   "A new proxy measure for health status." Paper presented at the American Public Health Association Meetings, Detroit, (November).

188. Klarman, H.E.
    1963   "Effect of prepaid group practice on hospital use." *Public Health Rep.* 17 (November): 955-965.

189. Klem, M.C.
    1965   "Physician services received in an urban community in relation to health insurance coverage." *Amer. J. Public Health* 55 (November): 1699-1716.

190. Knezo, G.J.
    1970   *The Social Sciences and Public Policy: A Selected Annotated Bibliography*. Washington: Library of Congress, Legislative Reference Service.

191. Knezo, G.J.
    1971   *Social Science Policies: An Annotated List of Recent Literature*. Washington: Library of Congress, Congressional Research Service.

192. Knezo, G.J.
    1973   *Social Indicators: A Review of Research and Policy Issues (Including Annotated Bibliography)*.

Washington: Library of Congress, Congressional Research Service.

193. Koos, E.L.
     1954   *The Health of Regionville.* New York: Columbia University Press.

194. Kovner, J.W.
     1969   "Measurement of outpatient office visit services." *Health Services Research* 4 (Summer): 112-127.

195. Kovner, J.W., et al.
     1969   "Income and the use of outpatient medical care by the insured." *Inquiry* 6 (June): 27-34.

196. Kriesberg, L.
     1963   "The relationship between socio-economic rank and behavior." *Social Problems* 10 (Spring): 334-352.

197. Kriesberg, L. and B.R. Treiman
     1960   "Socioeconomic status and utilization of dentists' services." *J. Amer. Coll. Dent.* 27 (September): 147-165.

198. Kriesberg, L. and B.R. Treiman
     1962   "Preventive utilization of dentists' services among teenagers." *J. Amer. Coll. Dent.* 29 (March): 28-45.

199. Land, K.C.
     1969   "Principles of path analysis." In Borgotta, F. (ed.), *Sociological Methodology, 1969.* San Francisco: Jossey Bass, Inc.

200. Land, K.C.
     1972   "Social indicator models: an overview." Unpub. manuscript. New York: Russell Sage Foundation and Columbia University.

201. Lavenhar, M.A., et al.
     1968   "Social class and medical care: indices of non-urgency in use of hospital emergency services." *Med. Care* 6 (September-October): 368-380.

202. Lefcowitz, M.J.
     1973   "Poverty and health: a re-examination." *Inquiry* 10 (March): 3-13.

203. Lerner, M.
1961   *Hospital Use by Diagnosis*. Research Series No. 16. Chicago: Center for Health Administration Studies, University of Chicago.

204. Lerner, M. and O.W. Anderson
1963   *Health Progress in the United States: 1900-1960*. Chicago: University of Chicago Press.

205. Levenson, I.
1972   "Access to medical care: the Queensbridge Experiment." *Inquiry* 9 (June): 61-68.

206. Li, F.P., et al.
1972   "Health care for the Chinese community in Boston." *Amer. J. Public Health* 62 (April): 536-539.

207. Lingoes, J.C. and M. Pfaff
1971   "Measurement of subjective welfare and satisfaction." Paper presented at the 84th Annual Meeting of the American Economic Association, New Orleans, Louisiana (December 27).

208. Lohr, W.
1972   "A historical view of the research done on the behavioral and organizational factors related to utilization of health services." Unpub. manuscript. National Center for Health Services Research and Development.

209. Lowenstein, R.
1971   "Early effects of Medicare on the health care of the aged." *Soc. Sec. Bull.* 34 (April): 3-20; 42.

210. Lowry, S., et al.
1958   "Factors associated with the acceptance of health care practices among rural families." *Rural Sociology* 23 (June): 198-202.

211. Ludwig, E.G. and G. Gibson
1969   "Self perception of sickness and the seeking of medical care." *J. Health Soc. Behav.* 10 (June): 125-133.

212. May, J.T.
1973   *Health Status: Health Action: Psycho-Social Indicators, Part II*. Nashville: Evaluation, Survey and Health Research Corporation.

213. Mechanic, D.
1972   *Public Expectations and Health Care: Essays on the Changing Organization of Health Services.* New York: John Wiley and Sons.

214. Meltzer, J.W. and J.R. Hochstim
1970   "Reliability and validity of survey data on physical health." *Public Health Rep.* 85 (December): 1075-1085.

215. Miller, M.H.
1973a   "Seeking advice for cancer symptoms." *Amer. J. Public Health* 63 (November): 955-961.

216. Miller, M.H.
1973b   "Who receives optimal medical care?" *J. Health Soc. Behav.* 14 (June). 176-182.

217. Mitchell, D.
1972   "Review of the literature on the use of health services." Unpub. manuscript. Washington: Institute of Medicine Health Services Research Study, National Academy of Sciences.

218. Montiero, L.A.
1973   "Expense is no object . . . income and physician visits reconsidered." *J. Health Soc. Behav.* 14 (June): 99-115.

219. Moore, G.T., et al.
1972   "Effect of a neighborhood health center on hospital emergency room use." *Med. Care* 2 (May-June): 240-247.

220. Moroney, R.M. and N. Kurtz
1973   "Extended care benefits: a comparison of utilization of two age groups." *Inquiry* 10 (March): 50-53.

221. Morris, N., et al.
1966a   "Alienation as a deterrent to well-child supervision." *Amer. J. Public Health* 56 (November): 1874-1882.

222. Morris, N., et al.
1966b   "Deterrents to well-child supervision." *Amer. J. Public Health* 56 (August): 1232-1241.

223. Mott, F.D., et al.
    1973   "Prepaid group practice in Sault Ste. Marie, Ontario: Part II. evidence from the household survey." *Med. Care* 11 (May-June): 173-188.

224. Muller, C.
    1965   "Income and the receipt of medical care." *Amer. J. Public Health* 55 (April): 510-521.

225. Murnaghan, J.H.
    1973   "Review of the Conference (on Ambulatory Medical Care Records) Proceedings." *Med. Care* 11 (March-April Supplement): 13-34.

226. McDonald, A.D., et al.
    1973   "Physician service in Montreal before universal health insurance." *Med. Care* 11 (July-August): 269-286.

227. McKinlay, J.B.
    1972   "Some approaches and problems in the study of the use of services — an overview." *J. Health Soc. Behav.* 13 (June): 115-152.

228. McKinley, J.B.
    1973   "Social networks, lay consultation and help-seeking behavior." *Social Forces* 51 (March): 275-292.

229. McKinlay, J.B. and S.M. McKinlay
    1972   "Some social characteristics of lower working class utilizers and underutilizers of maternity care services." *J. Health Soc. Behav.* 13 (December): 369-392.

230. McVeigh, T.
    1971   *Social Indicators: A Bibliography.* Monticello, Illinois: Council of Planning Librarians Exchange Bibliography #215.

National Center for Health Statistics
    Series 2

231.   1965a   *An Index of Health: Mathematical Models.* Number 5.

232.   1965b   *Health Interview Responses Compared with Medical Records.* Number 7.

233.   1966   *Conceptual Problems in Developing an Index of Health.* Number 17.

234.   1967   *Interview Data on Chronic Conditions Compared with Information Derived from Medical Records.* Number 23.

235.   1969   *International Comparisons of Medical Care Utilization.* Number 33.

236.   1971   *Disability Components for an Index of Health.* Number 42.

237.   1972a   *Interviewing Methods in the Health Interview Survey.* Number 48.

238.   1972b   *Reporting Health Events in Household Interviews: Effects of an Extensive Questionnaire on a Diary Procedure.* Number 49.

239.   1973   *Net Differences in Interview Data on Chronic Conditions and Information Derived from Medical Records.* Number 57.

Series 10

240.   1963   *Family Income in Relation to Selected Health Characteristics.* Number 2.

241.   1964a   *Current Estimates from the Health Interview Survey: United States —July 1962-June 1963.* Number 5.

242.   1964b   *Medical Care, Health Status and Family Income: United States — 1963.* Number 9.

243.   1964c   *Current Estimates from the Health Interview Survey: United States —July 1963-June 1964.* Number 13.

244.   1965a   *Volume of Physician Visits by Place of Visit, and Type of Service: United States — July 1957-June 1964.* Number 18.

245.   1965b   *Physician Visits —Interval of Visits and Children's Routine Checkup: United States — July 1963-June 1964.* Number 19.

246. 1965c *Persons Hospitalized by Number of Hospital Episodes and Days in a Year: United States — July 1960-June 1962.* Number 20.

247. 1965d *Personal Health Expenses: Distribution of Persons by Amount and Type of Expense: United States — July-December 1962.* Number 22.

248. 1965e *Volume of Dental Visits: United States — July 1963-June 1964.* Number 23.

249. 1966a *Personal Health Expenses — Per Capita Annual Expenses: United States — July-December 1962.* Number 27.

250. 1966b *Dental Visits — Time Interval Since Last Visit: United States — July 1963-June 1964.* Number 29.

251. 1966c *Hospital Discharges and Length of Stay: Short-Stay Hospitals: United States — July 1963-June 1964.* Number 30.

252. 1966d *Age Patterns in Medical Care, Illness and Disability: United States — July 1963-June 1965.* Number 32.

253. 1966e *Cost and Acquisitions of Prescribed and Nonprescribed Medicines: United States — July 1964-June 1965.* Number 33.

254. 1967a *Health Characteristics by Geographic Region, Large Metropolitan Areas, and Other Places of Residence: United States — July 1963-June 1965.* Number 36.

255. 1967b *Current Estimates from the Health Interview Survey: United States — July 1965-June 1966.* Number 37.

256. 1967c *Prescribed and Non-prescribed Medicine: Type and Use of Medicines: United States — July 1964-June 1965.* Number 39.

257. 1968a *Current Estimates from the Health Interview Survey: United States — July 1966-June 1967.* Number 43.

258.   1968b   *Volume of Physician Visits: United States — July 1966-June 1967.* Volume 49.

259.   1969a   *Persons Hospitalized by Number of Hospital Illness Episodes and Days in a Year: United States — July 1965-June 1966.* Number 50.

260.   1969b   *Characteristics of Persons with Corrective Lenses: United States — July 1965-June 1966.* Number 53.

261.   1969c   *Family Use of Health Services: United States — July 1963-June 1964.* Number 55.

262.   1969d   *Differentials in Health Characteristics by Color: United States — July 1965-June 1967.* Number 56.

263.   1970   *Current Estimates from the Health Interview Survey: United States — 1968.* Number 60.

264.   1971a   *Children and Youth — Selected Health Characteristics: United States — 1958 and 1968.* Number 62.

265.   1971b   *Current Estimates from the Health Interview Survey: United States — 1969.* Number 63.

266.   1971c   *Persons Hospitalized by Number of Hospital Episodes and Days in a Year: United States — 1968.* Number 64.

267.   1972a   *Hospital and Surgical Insurance Coverage: United States — 1968.* Number 66.

268.   1972b   *Disability Days: United States — 1968.* Number 67.

269.   1972c   *Age Patterns in Medical Care, Illness and Disability: United States, 1968-1969.* Number 70.

270.   1972d   *Current Estimates from the Health Interview Survey: United States — 1970.* Number 72.

271.   1972e   *Home Care for Persons 55 Years and Over: United States — July 1966-June 1968.* Number 73.

272.   1972f   *Health Characteristics of Low-Income Persons.* Number 74.

273.   1972g   *Physician Visits: Volume and Interval Since Last Visit: United States — 1969.* Number 75.

274.   1972h   *Dental Visits: Volume and Interval Since Last Visit: United States — 1969.* Number 76.

275.   1972i   *Acute Conditions: Incidence and Associated Disability: United States — July 1969-June 1970.* Number 77.

276.   1972j   *Use of Special Aids: United States —1969.* Number 78.

277.   1973a   *Current Estimates from the Health Interview Survey: United States — 1971.* Number 79.

278.   1973b   *Volume of X-Ray Visits: United States — April-September 1970.* Number 81.

Series 12

279.   1965a   *Characteristics of Residents in Institutions for the Aged and Chronically Ill.* Number 2.

280.   1965b   *Characteristics of Patients in Mental Hospitals: United States — April-June 1973.* Number 3.

281.   1966   *Utilization of Institutions for the Aged and Chronically Ill: United States —April-June 1963.* Number 4.

282.   1967a   *Chronic Illness Among Residents of Nursing and Personal Care Homes: United States — May-June 1964.* Number 7.

283.   1967b   *Prevalence of Chronic Conditions and Impairments Among Residents of Nursing and Personal Care Homes: United States — May-June 1964.* Number 8.

284.   1968a   *Nursing and Personal Care Services Received by Residents of Nursing and Personal Care Homes: United States — May-June 1964.* Number 10.

285.   1968b   *Use of Special Aids in Homes for the Aged and Chronically Ill: United States — May-June, 1964.* Number 11.

286.   1969   *Marital Status and Living Arrangements Before Admission to Nursing and Personal Care Homes: United States — May-June 1964.* Number 12.

287.   1970   *Arrangements for Physician Services to Residents in Nursing and Personal Care Homes: United States — May-June 1964.* Number 13.

288.   1972a   *Nursing Homes: Their Admission Policies, Admissions, and Discharges: United States — April-September 1968.* Number 16.

289.   1972b   *Services and Activities Offered to Nursing Home Residents: United States — 1968.* Number 17.

290.   1973a   *Characteristics of Residents in Nursing and Personal Care Homes: United States — June-August 1969.* Number 19.

291.   1973b   *Charges for Care and Sources of Payment for Residents in Nursing Homes: United States — June-August 1969.* Number 21.

Series 13

292.   1966   *Patients Discharged from Short-Stay Hospitals: United States — October-December 1964.* Number 1.

293.   1967a   *Utilization of Short-Stay Hospitals — Summary of Non-medical Statistics: United States — 1965.* Number 2.

294.   1967b   *Utilization of Short-Stay Hospitals by Characteristics of Discharged Patients: United States — 1965.* Number 3.

295.   1968   *Patients Discharged from Short-Stay Hospitals by Size and Type of Ownership: United States — 1965.* Number 4.

296.   1969   *Regional Utilization of Short-Stay Hospitals: United States — 1965.* Number 5.

297.   1970   *Inpatient Utilization of Short-Stay Hospitals by Diagnosis: United States — 1965.* Number 6.

298.   1971   *Utilization of Short-Stay Hospitals: Summary of Nonmedical Statistics: United States — 1966.* Number 8.

299.　1972a　*Utilization of Short-Stay Hospitals: Summary of Nonmedical Statistics: United States — 1967.* Number 9.

300.　1972b　*Inpatient Utilization of Short-Stay Hospitals in Each Geographic Region: United States — 1966-1968.* Number 10.

301.　1973a　*Inpatient Utilization of Short-Stay Hospitals by Diagnosis: United States — 1968.* Number 12.

302.　1973b　*Average Length of Stay in Short-Stay Hospitals — Demographic Factors: United States — 1968.* Number 13.

303.　1973c　*Utilization of Short-Stay Hospitals — Summary of Nonmedical Statistics: United States — 1970.* Number 14.

Series 22

304.　1968a　*Visits for Medical and Dental Care During the Year Preceding Childbirth: United States — 1963 Births.* Number 4.

305　1968　*Medical X-ray Visits and Examinations During Pregnancy: United States — 1963.* Number 5.

306. Newman, J.
　1973　"Problems in the development of indicators of health status: some demographic considerations." Paper presented at Population Association of America meetings, New Orleans (April 25-28).

307. Newman, J. and O.W. Anderson
　1972　*Patterns of Dental Services Utilization in the United States: A Nationwide Social Survey. Research Series No. 30.* Chicago: Center for Health Administration Studies, University of Chicago.

308. Nikias, M.K.
　1968　"Social class and the use of dental care under prepayment." *Med. Care* 6 (September-October): 381-393.

309. Noble, J.H., et al.
     1971   "Variations in visits to hospital emergency care
               facilities: ritualistic and meteorological factors af-
               fecting supply and demand." *Med. Care* 9
               (September-October): 415-427.

310. Nolan, R.L., et al.
     1967   "Social class differences in utilization of pediatric
               services in a prepaid direct service medical care pro-
               gram." *Amer. J. Public Health* 57 (January): 34-47.

311. Nyman, K. and E. Kalimo
     1973   "National sickness insurance and the use of physi-
               cians' services in Finland." *Soc. Sci. Med.* 7 (July):
               541-553.

312. Olendzki, M.C., et al.
     1972   "The impact of Medicaid on private care for the
               urban poor." *Med. Care* 10 (May-June): 201-206.

313. O'Shea, R.M. and G.D. Bissell
     1969   "Dental services under Medicaid: the experience of
               Erie County, New York" *Amer. J. Public Health* 59
               (May): 832-840.

314. Palmore, E. and C. Luikart
     1972   "Health and social factors related to life satisfac-
               tion." *J. Health Soc. Behav.* 13 (March): 68-80.

315. Passman, M.J.
     1966   "Hospital utilization by Blue Cross members in 1964
               according to selected demographic and enrollment
               characteristics." *Inquiry* 3 (May): 82-89.

316. Patrick, D.L., et al.
     1973   "Toward an operational definition of health." *J.
               Health Soc. Behav.* 14 (March): 6-23.

317. Perrott, G.S.
     1971   "The federal employees health benefits program:
               enrollment and utilization of health services —
               1961-1968." Washington: U.S. Govt. Printing Of-
               fice.

318. Peterson, M.L.
     1971   "The first year in Columbia: assessments of low
               hospitalization rate and high office use." *Johns
               Hopkins Med. J.* 128 (January): 15-23.

319. Pettengill, J.H.
    1972   "Trends in hospital use by the aged." *Soc. Sec. Bull.*
            35 (July): 3-15.

320. Phelps, C.E. and J.P. Newhouse
    1972   "Effect of coinsurance: a multivariate analysis."
            Soc. Sec. Bull. 35 (June): 20-28;44.

321. Picken, B. and G. Ireland
    1969   "Family patterns of medical care utilization: possi-
            ble influences of family size, role and social class on
            illness behavior." *J. Chronic Dis.* 22 (August):
            181-191.

322. Podell, L.
    1969   *Studies on the Use of Health Services by Families
            on Welfare: Utilization of Preventive Health Ser-
            vices (Supplementary Report).* New York: The
            Center for the Study of Urban Problems, Bernard
            M. Baruch College, The City University of New
            York.

323. Pomeroy, R., et al.
    1970   *Studies on the Use of Health Services by Families
            on Welfare: Utilization by Publicly-Assisted
            Families.* New York: The Center for the Study of
            Urban Problems, Bernard M. Baruch College, The
            City University of New York.

324. Pope, C.R., et al.
    1969   "Determinants of medical care utilization: the use of
            the telephone for reporting symptoms." *J. Health
            Soc. Behav.* 12 (June): 155-162.

325. Purola, T.
    1973   *Health Insurance, the Incidence of Illness, and the
            Use of Medical Services.* Unpub. manuscript. Hel-
            sinki: Research Institute for Social Security.

326. Purola, T., et al.
    1968   *The Utilization of Medical Services and its Rela-
            tionship to Morbidity, Health Resources and Social
            Factors.* Helsinki: Research Institute for Social
            Security.

327. Rabin, D.L.
    1972   "International comparisons of medical care." *Milb.
            Mem. Fund Quart.* 50 (July): 1-99.

328. Rayner, J.F.
      1970   "Socioeconomic status and factors influencing the dental health practices of mothers." *Amer. J. Public Health* 60 (July): 1250-1257.

329. Redick, R.
      1971   *1970 Census Data Used to Indicate Areas with Different Potentials for Mental Health and Related Problems.* No. 3 of Series C, "Mental Health Statistics," National Institute of Mental Health Services. Public Health Service Publication No. 2171. Washington: U.S. Govt. Printing Office.

330. Reed, L.S. and W. Carr
      1968   "Utilization and cost of general hospital care: Canada and the United States, 1948-1966." *Soc. Sec. Bull.* 31 (November): 12-20.

331. Regional Medical Programs Service
      1973   *Quality Assurance of Medical Care.* Monograph, Washington: U.S. Dept. HEW.

332. Rein, M.
      1969   "Social class and the utilization of medical care services: a study of British experience under the National Health Service." *Hospitals* 43 (July 1): 43-54.

333. Reinke, W.A., and T.D. Baker
      1967   "Measuring effects of demographic variables on health services utilization." *Health Services Research* 2 (Spring): 61-75.

334. Richards, N.D.
      1971   "Utilization of dental services." In Richards, N.D. and L.K. Cohen (eds.), *Social Sciences and Dentistry: A Critical Bibliography.* The Hague, Netherlands: Federation Dentaire Internationale.

335. Richardson, A.H. and H.E. Freeman
      1969   "Use of extended health benefit program by octogenarian U.A.W. retireees." *Med. Care* 7 (May-June): 225-234.

336. Richardson, A.H. and H.E. Freeman
      1972   "Evaluation of medical care utilization by interview surveys." *Med. Care* 10 (July-August): 357-362.

337. Richardson, A.H., et al.
     1967   "Use of medical resources by SPANCOS: II. So-
             cial factors and medical care experience." *Milb.
             Mem. Fund Quart.* 45 (January): 61-75.

338. Richardson, F.M.
     1972   "Peer review of medical care." *Med. Care* 10
             (January-February): 29-39.

339. Richardson, J.D. and F.D. Scutchfield
     1973   "Priorities in health care: the consumer's viewpoint
             in an Appalachian community." *Amer. J. Public
             Health* 63 (January): 79-82.

340. Richardson, W.C.
     1969   "Poverty, illness and use of health services in the
             United States." *Hospitals* 43 (July 1): 34-40.

341. Richardson, W.C.
     1970   "Measuring the urban poor's use of physicians ser-
             vices in response to illness episodes." *Med. Care* 8
             (March-April): 132-142.

342. Richardson, W.C.
     1971   *Ambulatory Use of Physician's Services in Re-
             sponse to Illness Episodes in a Low-Income Neigh-
             borhood.* Research Series No. 29. Chicago: Center
             for Health Administration Studies, University of
             Chicago.

343. Robertson, R.L.
     1972   "Comparative medical care use under prepaid group
             practice and free choice plans: a case study."
             Inquiry 9 (September): 70-76.

344. Robinson, G.C., et al.
     1969   "Use of a hospital emergency service by children
             and adolescents for primary care." *Canada Med.
             Assoc. J.* 101 (November 1): 69-73.

345. Robinson, W.S.
     1950   "Ecological correlations and the behavior of indi-
             viduals." *ASR* 15 (June): 351-357.

346. Rodman, A.
     1965   "Comparison of Baltimore's utilization rates under
             two physician-payment systems." *Public Health
             Rep.* 80 (June): 476-480.

347. Roemer, M.I.
     1958   "Influence of prepaid physician's services on hospi-
               tal utilization. *Hospitals* 32 (October 16): 48-52.

348. Roemer, M.I.
     1961a   "Bed supply and hospital utilization." *Hospitals* 35
               (November 1): 36-42.

349. Roemer, M.I.
     1961b   "Hospital utilization and the supply of physicians."
               JAMA 178 (December 9): 987-993.

350. Rogers, D.E.
     1973   "Shattuck lecture — the American health-care
               scene." *New Eng. J. Med.* 288 (June 28): 1377-1383.

351. Roghmann, K.J. and R.J. Haggerty
     1970   "The utilization of child health services: distribu-
               tions, patterns, and barriers." Unpub. manuscript.
               Rochester, New York: University of Rochester.

352. Roghmann, K.J., et al.
     1970a   "Anticipated and actual effects of Medicaid on the
               care pattern of children." Unpub. manuscript.
               Rochester, New York: University of Rochester.

353. Roghmann, K.J., et al.
     1970b   "Child health services: volume and flow in a met-
               ropolitan community." Unpub. manuscript.
               Rochester, New York: University of Rochester.

354. Roos, N.P.
     1973   "Evaluating the impact of health programs: moving
               from here to there." Paper presented at Workshop,
               Center for Health Administration Studies, Chicago
               (October 11).

355. Rosenblatt, D. and E. Suchman
     1964   "The underutilization of medical-care services by
               the blue-collarites." In Shostak, A. and W. Gom-
               berg (eds.), *Blue-Collar World*. Englewood Cliffs:
               Prentice-Hall.

356. Rosenstock, I.M.
     1966   "Why people use health services." *Milb. Mem.
               Fund Quart.* 44 (July): 94-127.

357. Rosenstock, I.M., et al.
     1959   "Why people fail to seek poliomyelitis vaccination."
               Public Health Rep. 74 (February): 98-103.

358. Rosenthal, G.
     1968   "Price elasticity of demand for short-term general
               hospital services." In Klarman, H.E. (ed.),
               Empirical Studies in Health Economics. Baltimore:
               The Johns Hopkins Press.

359. Ross, J.A.
     1962   "Social class and medical care." *J. Health Hum.
               Behav.* 4 (Spring): 35-40.

360. Roth, J.A.
     1971   "Utilization of the hospital emergency depart-
               ment." *J. Health Soc. Behav.* 12 (December):
               312-320.

361. Salber, E.J., et al.
     1971   "Utilization of services at a neighborhood health
               center." *Pediatrics* 47 (February): 415-423.

362. Sanders, B.S.
     1964   "Measuring community health levels." *Amer. J.
               Public Health* 54 (July): 1063-1070.

363. Satin, D.G.
     1973   " 'Help': the hospital emergency unit patient and his
               presenting picture." *Med. Care* 11 (July-August):
               328-337.

364. Satin, D.G. and F.J. Duhl
     1972   "Help?: the hospital emergency unit as community
               physician." *Med. Care* 10 (May-June): 248-260.

364. Schoen, M.H.
     1973   "Observation of selected dental services under two
               prepayment mechanisms." *Amer. J. Public Health*
               63 (August): 727-731.

366. Schonfeld, H.K.
     1968   "The development of standards for the audit and
               planning of medical care: audit of hospital outpatient
               care." Paper presented at the Conference on Audit-
               ing Outpatient Care, Minneapolis (March 29).

152   *Access to Medical Care*

367. Schonfeld, H.K.
     1970   "Standards for the audit and planning of medical
                 care: a method for preparing audit standards for mix-
                 tures of patients." *Med. Care* 8 (July-August):
                 287-298.

368. Schonfeld, H.K., et al.
     1967   "The content of good dental care: methodology in a
                 formulation for clinical standards and audits, and
                 preliminary findings." *Amer. J. Public Health* 57
                 (July): 1137-1146.

369. Schonfeld, H.K., et al.
     1968a   "The development of standards for the audit and
                 planning of medical care: good pediatric care — pro-
                 gram content and method of estimating needed per-
                 sonnel." *Amer. J. Public Health* 58 (November):
                 2097-2110.

370. Schonfeld, H.K., et al.
     1968b   "The development of standards for the audit and
                 planning of medical care: pathways among primary
                 physicians and specialists for diagnosis and treat-
                 ment." *Med. Care* 6 (March-April): 110-114.

371. Schonfeld, H.K., et al.
     1972   "Number of physicians required for primary medi-
                 cal care." *New Eng. J. Med.* 286 (March 16):
                 571-576.

372. Schonfield, J., et al.
     1963   "Medical attitudes and practices of parents toward a
                 mass tuberculin testing program." *Amer. J. Public
                 Health* 53 (May): 772-781.

373. Schneider, G.E. and S. Fox
     1973   "Health care coverage and out-of-pocket expendi-
                 tures of Detroit families." *Inquiry* 10 (December):
                 49-57.

374. Schragg, H., et al.
     1973   "Low income families in a large prepaid group prac-
                 tice." *Inquiry* 10 (June): 52-60.

375. Scitovsky, A.A. and N.M. Snyder
     1972   "Effect of coinsurance on use of physician ser-
                 vices." *Soc. Sec. Bull.* 35 (June): 3-19.

376. Shain, M.
1968   "Hospital admission rates under Medicare and the former OAA medical program." *Inquiry* 5 (March): 65-67.

377. Shain, M. and M.I. Roemer
1959   "Hospital costs relate to supply of beds." *Mod. Hosp.* 92 (April): 71-73.

378. Shanas, E.
1960   *Medical Care Among Those Aged 65 and Over.* Research Series No. 16. Chicago: Center for Health Administration Studies, University of Chicago.

379. Shannon, G.W., et al.
1969   "The concept of distance as a factor in accessibility and utilization of health care." *Med. Care Rev.* 26 (February): 143-161.

380. Shannon, G.W., et al.
1973   "Time and distance: the journey for medical care." *Intl. J. Health Services* 3 (Spring): 237-243.

381. Shapiro, S.
1967   "Patterns of medical use by the indigent aged under two systems of medical care." *Amer. J. Public Health* 57 (May): 784-790.

382. Shapiro, S. and J. Brindle
1969   "Serving Medicaid eligibles." *Amer. J. Public Health* 59 (April): 635-641.

383. Sheldon, E.B. and H. Freeman
1970   "Notes on social indicators: promises and potentials." *Policy Sciences* 1 (Spring): 97-111.

384. Shortell, S.
1972   *A Model of Physician Referral Behavior: A Test of Exchange Theory in Medical Practice.* Research Series No. 31. Chicago: Center for Health Administration Studies, University of Chicago.

385. Shortell, S.
1973   "Patterns of medical care: issues of access, cost, and continuity." Paper presented at Workshop, Center for Health Administration Studies, Chicago (April 5).

386. Shortell, S. and O.W. Anderson
  1971   "The physician referral process: a theoretical pers-
            pective." *Health Services Research* 6 (Spring):
            39-48.

387. Sills, D.L. and R.E. Gill
  1958   "Young adults' use of the Salk vaccine." *Social
            Problems* 6 (Winter): 246-253.

388. Simon, J.L. and D.B. Smith
  1973   "Change in location of a student health service: a
            quasi-experimental evaluation of the effects of dis-
            tance on utilization." *Med. Care* 11 (January-
            February): 59-67.

389. Social Science Research Council
  1973   Social Indicators Newsletters (current issues).

390. Solon, J.A.
  1966   "Patterns of medical care: sociocultural variations
            among a hospital's outpatients." *Amer. J. Public
            Health* 55 (June): 884-894.

391. Solon, J.A. and R.D. Rigg
  1972   "Patterns of medical care among users of hospital
            emergency units." *Med. Care* 10 (January-
            February): 60-72.

392. Solon, J.A., et al.
  1967   "Delineating episodes of medical care." *Amer. J.
            Public Health* 57 (March): 401-408.

393. Solon, J.A., et al.
  1969   "Episodes of medical care: nursing students' use of
            medical services." *Amer. J. Public Health* 59 (June):
            936-946.

394. Somers, A.R.
  1971   *Health Care in Transition: Directions for the Fu-
            ture.* Chicago: Hospital Research and Educational
            Trust.

395. Somers, H.M. and A.R. Somers
  1961   *Doctors, Patients and Health Insurance.*
            Washington: The Brookings Institution.

396. Sparer, G. and A. Anderson
1973   "Utilization and cost experience of low-income families in four prepaid group-practice plans." *New Eng. J. Med.* 289 (July 12): 67-72.

397. Sparer, G. and L. Okada
1971   "Differential patterns of poverty and health care utilization in eight urban areas." Paper presented at the meetings of the American Association of Public Opinion Research, Pasadena, California (May 22).

398. Stanford Research Institute
1969   *Toward Master Social Indicators.* Research Memorandum EPRC-6747-2. Menlo Park: SRI.

399. Steele, J.L. and W.H. McBroom
1972   "Conceptual and empirical dimensions of health behavior." *J. Health Soc. Behav.* 13 (December): 382-392.

400. Stine, O., et al.
1968   "Broken appointments at a comprehensive child clinic for children." *Med. Care* 6 (July-August): 332-339.

401. Strauss, M.A. and G. Sparer
1971   "Basic utilization experience of OEO comprehensive health service projects." *Inquiry* 8 (December): 36-49.

402. Suchman, E.
1965   "Social patterns of illness and medical care." *J. Health Hum. Behav.* 6 (Spring): 2-16.

403. Teller, C.H.
1973   "Access to medical care of migrants in a Honduran city." *J. Health Soc. Behav.* 14 (September): 214-226.

404. Torrens, P.R. and D.G. Yedvab
1970   "Variations among emergency room populations: a comparison of four hospitals in New York City." *Med. Care* 8 (January-February): 60-75.

405. Tyroler, H., et al.
1965   "Patterns of preventive health behavior in populations." *J. Health Hum. Behav.* 6 (Fall): 128-140.

406. U.S. Department of Agriculture
1973   *Health Services in Rural America.* Agriculture Information Bulletin No. 362. Washington: U.S. Department of Agriculture, Rural Development Service.

407. U.S. Department of Health, Education and Welfare
1969   *Toward a Social Report.* Washington: U.S. Govt. Printing Office.

408. U.S. Public Health Service
1958   *Public Participation in Medical Screening Programs: A Socio-psychological Study.* PHS No. 572. Washington: U.S. Govt. Printing Office.

409. U.S. Public Health Service.
1959   *Dental Care in a Group Purchase Plan: A Survey of Attitudes and Utilization in the St. Louis Labor Health Institute.* PHS No. 684. Washington: U.S. Govt. Printing Office.

410. U.S. Public Health Service
1969a   *Population Characteristics and Participation in the Poliomyelitis Vaccination Program.* PHS No. 723. Washington: U.S. Govt. Printing Office.

411. U.S. Public Health Service
1969b   *Proceedings of a Conference on Conceptual Issues in the Analysis of Medical Care Utilization Behavior.* Conference Sponsored by Kaiser Foundation Hospitals and National Center for Health Services Research and Development, Portland, Oregon (October).

412. VanDyke, F. and V. Brown
1972   "Organized home care: an alternative to institutions." *Inquiry* 9 (June): 3-16.

413. Voorhis, G.
1972   "The health services system in the United States: a review of the literature." Unpub. manuscript. Chicago: Center for Health Administration Studies, University of Chicago.

414. Watkins, E.
1968   "Low-income Negro mothers: their decision to seek prenatal care." *Amer. J. Public Health* 58 (April): 655-667.

415. Weinerman, E.R., et al.
    1966   "Yale studies in ambulatory medical care: V. Determinants of use of hospital emergency services." *Amer. J. Public Health* 56 (July): 1037-1056.

416. Weiss, G.L.
    1972   "The influence of need for care and selected sociodemographic characteristics on the utilization of physician services." Unpub. M.S. thesis. Lafayette, Indiana: Department of Sociology, Purdue University.

417. Weiss, J.E. and M.R. Greenlick
    1970   "Determinants of medical care utilization: the effect of social class and distance on contacts with the medical care system." *Med. Care* 8 (November-December): 456-462.

418. Weiss, J.E., et al.
    1971   "Determinants of medical care utilization: the impact of spatial factors." *Inquiry* 8 (December): 50-57.

419. Welch, S., et al.
    1973   "Some social and attitudinal correlates of health care among Mexican-Americans." *J. Health Soc. Behav.* 14 (September): 205-213.

420. White, E.L.
    1968   "A graphic presentation on age and income differentials in selected aspects of morbidity, disability and utilization of health services." *Inquiry* 5 (March): 18-30.

421. White, H.A., et al.
    1970   "Use of the emergency room in a community hospital." *Public Health Rep.* 85 (February): 163-168.

422. Wilcox, L.D., et al.
    1972   *Social Indicators and Societal Monitoring: An Annotated Bibliography.* San Francisco: Jossey-Bass, Inc.

423. Williams, R.
    1966   "A comparison of hospital utilization and costs by types of coverage." *Inquiry* 3 (September): 28-42.

424. Wingert, W.A., et al.
     1968   "The influence of family organization on the utiliza-
               tion of pediatric emergency services." *Pediatrics* 42
               (November): 743-751.

425. Winkelstein, W., Jr. and S. Graham
     1959   "Factors in participation in the 1954 poliomyelitis
               vaccine field trials, Erie County, New York."
               Amer. J. Public Health 49 (November): 1454-1466.

426. Wirick, G.C., Jr.
     1962a   "A multiple equation model of demand for health
               care." *Health Services Research* 1 (Winter):
               301-346.

427. Wirick, G.C., Jr.
     1962b   "Population survey: health care and its financing."
               In McNerney, W.J., et al. *Hospital and Medical
               Economics.* Chicago: Hospital Research and Edu-
               cational Trust.

428. Wolfe, S. and R.F. Badgley
     1972   "The family doctor." *Milb. Mem. Fund Quart.* 50
               (April): 1-203.

429. Yankauer, A., et al.
     1953   "An evaluation of prenatal care and its relationship
               to social class and social disorganization." *Amer. J.
               Public Health* 43 (August): 1001-1010.

430. Yankauer, A., et al.
     1958   "Social stratification and health practices in child-
               bearing and childrearing." *Amer. J. Public Health*
               48 (June): 732-741.

431. Yeracaris, C.
     1962   "Social factors associated with the acceptance of
               medical innovations: a pilot study." *J. Health Hum.
               Behav.* 3 (Fall): 193-198.

432. Zola, I.K.
     1966   "Culture and symptoms — an analysis of patients'
               presenting complaints." *ASR* 31 (October): 615-630.

5

Selected Abstracts

Introduction

These abstracts report the purpose, population and/or sample and method of data collection, process and outcome indices of access, method of data analysis and findings for each reference. The emphasis was on abstracting empirical articles. Some few theoretical books and articles were also included, however. This selection of abstracts serves to update a bibliography on the indices and correlates of health services utilization, published in early 1972 (Aday and Eichhorn, 1972).

ABSTRACTS

Abernathy, W.J. and J.R. Moore

>1972   "Regional planning of primary health care services." *Med. Care.* 10 (September-October): 380-394.

The purpose of this study is to describe a method of approach to utilization analysis that can provide insights to health policy formulation on a community or regional basis.

The study surveyed families in widely diverse socioeconomic groups in a well-defined agricultural region 100 miles from San Francisco in the San Joaquin Valley. A special census provided socio-demographic information on the population.

The utilization index was the deviation from the national average of the percent of family members that visited a physician in the past year. It was computed as follows: $U = n\text{-}a/k$, where "n" = number of family members who saw a physician in the past year; "a" = average or expected number of family members who saw a doctor during the period (derived from National Center for Health Statistics data); and "k" = size of the family.

The variables used in AID analysis to construct statistically homogeneous use sub-groups or strata were residency duration, industry of employment, occupation, education, ethnicity, religion, income and source of medical payment. The independent variables considered in multiple regression analysis within each stratum were income, education, age, language, distance from the facility and residency duration.

The AID analysis permits identification of a number of groups or clusters within the community that are relatively homogeneous in their utilization behavior — short-term resident Mexican-Americans, residents three years or more, laborers, etc. The impact of selected socioeconomic factors on utilization within each of these strata is evaluated using stepwise regression analysis. Language is a significant barrier to utilization for Japanese-American and Portuguese families. An inverse effect of income on use was found for Medi-Cal recipients. The relationships of residency, travel time, etc. for the different strata are also reported.

Acton, J.P.

1972   "Demand for health care among the urban poor, with special emphasis on the role of time." Unpub. manuscript. Santa Monica, California: Rand Corporation.

This study analyzes the impact of factors, such as waiting or travel times on the urban poor's demand for medical care, as prices become less significant, due to the advent of universal health insurance coverage.

Data came from the OEO neighborhood health center baseline surveys in Red Hook and Bedford-Crown-Stuyvesant, New York.

The utilization indices examined were number of visits in the past year to physician in hospital outpatient or other clinic and to a physician in his private office; number of days hospitalized in city or governmental hospital and number of days in non-governmental hospitals.

The variables used to predict demand were age, sex, race, education, family size, income, insurance coverage, price, travel time, waiting time and number of chronic conditions limiting activity.

Tobit analysis was used to estimate the coefficients of a series of multivariate equations.

The author presented a utility maximization model that predicted that demand for medical services will become more sensitive to changes in travel and waiting time as the money prices shrink due to spreading insurance coverage. The findings seemed to confirm this hypothesis. For the populations studied, the majority of whom have "free" insurance through Medicaid and/or Medicare, demand for care was more sensitive to variation in "time prices" than to money prices of medical services. Race and health status also had significant effects on demand for medical services.

The author discusses the implications of these findings, e.g., 1) time may replace money as the rationing mechanism of demand under National Health Insurance; 2) to increase medical access, reducing travel and waiting time are important aspects to consider; and 3) to increase access by the poor, it may be important to consider income subsidy rather than direct medical subsidy to the poor.

Aday, L.A.

    1973   "Economic and non-economic barriers to the use of needed medical services." Unpub. Ph.D. dissertation. Lafayette, Indiana: Department of Sociology, Purdue University.

This study introduces a use-disability ratio, to monitor peoples' access to the use of needed medical services.

Data came from the 1971 CHAS-NORC national survey of health services utilization.

The use-disability ratio was constructed by dividing the mean physician visits in two weeks for those who had one or more disability days by their mean disability days and multiplying by 100. "Appropriate", "under", and "over" utilizers were identified by whether or not those with (and without) disability days contacted a physician.

The indices were analyzed for the following variables: age, sex, race, education, usual source of care, time to usual source of care, poverty level and insurance coverage.

Cross-tabulation of rates was used to analyze the data.

The article points out how considering use and need together, in terms of the use-disability ratio, yields different results than looking simply at volume of visits alone, as is done in much of the literature. The use of services, relative to need by the elderly, is less than other age groups, though their mean number of visits is higher. Males and females had similar scores on the ratio, though women consistently report more total contacts with a physician. The use of needed services for nonwhites for whom the economic barriers are minimized (the nonpoor insured) actually average more visits than whites. The poorly-educated average fewer visits, relative to need, than the best-educated. Whether or not one has a usual source of care and the distance to this source appear to make little difference with respect to who gets care when the need arises.

Though the poor now average more physician visits than the nonpoor, their use, relative to need, is still less than the well-to-do. The findings for the use-disability ratio show that the use of services relative to need is not noticeably increased by insurance for those groups that have been the special targets of programs to eliminate the economic barriers to access through third-party coverage — the poor, nonwhites, and the elderly.

Albrecht, S.L. and M.K. Miller

     1973   "Health service delivery: an assessment of some adequacy indicators." Paper presented at the Rural Sociology Society meetings, Baltimore (August).

The purpose of this paper is to demonstrate the impact of the existence of service delivery units on people's satisfaction with the adequacy of their medical care.

Data presented came from two sources: 1) published data from secondary sources, such as the report entitled "Utah health facts," and Bureau of the Census publications; and 2) survey interview data collected from random samples in three rural Utah counties (Wayne, Piute, and Beaver) and one urban county (Salt Lake).

Measures of consumer satisfaction included the number of miles reported that one must travel to get "adequate" health facilities, willingness to pay increased taxes to provide better health and medical services, percent who would visit a doctor more often if he were readily available, percent needing medical services not received, and stage of illness at which doctor is consulted.

The spatial distribution of hospitals and physicians — number of hospitals and number of physicians per 100 square miles — is used as a service adequacy indicator in the diffferent counties. The rural counties have much lower ratios than urban Salt Lake County.

Cross-tabulation of rates and percentages and correlation analysis were used to analyze the data.

The authors argue that a distributional variable, such as number of medical service units per 100 square miles, is a much better index of the *quality* of medical care available in an area than population-based measures, such as physicians per 1,000. The rank order correlations, for example, were found to be much higher between selected socio-economic variables (percent of county's population in professional occupations, percent urban, median family income, etc.) and hospitals and physicians per 100 square miles than between these same variables and hospitals and physicians per 1,000 population.

In the counties studied, the rural counties appeared to be at a much greater disadvantage with respect to service adequacy using the spatial, rather than the population-based resource availability ratios. The "perceived" adequacy of services on the part of residents in the rural counties was also found to be much less than in the urban county. A much larger percent of rural residents reported having to travel more than 25 miles to get adequate care. Over 95 percent of the residents of the two rural counties where there were no hospitals or physicians rated their community's medical facilities "poor." People in the most disadvantaged rural counties were more willing to pay increased taxes for improved medical services than for any other service. Over 50 percent said they would visit a doctor more often if one were readily available (compared to 12.1 percent in urban county). The percent who reported needing medical services, but had not received any, was higher in the rural counties. Over 50 percent of the residents of the two most disadvantaged rural counties said they saw a doctor only when absolutely necessary, compared to 29.8 percent in the urban county.

Alpert, J.J., et al.

1970   "Attitudes and satisfaction of low-income families receiving comprehensive pediatric care." *Amer. J. Public Health* 60 (March): 499-506.

The purpose of this study is to evaluate the attitudes of low-income families toward a program of comprehensive health care for their children and to determine if they are satisfied with the new program.

Seven hundred and fifty (750) low-income families who used the Boston Children's Hospital Medical Center Emergency Clinic, lived within three miles of the clinic and had no regular family physician constituted the sample. The sample was randomly assigned to an experimental group who received "comprehensive, family-focused pediatric care" for three years. The remainder were assigned to an "attention-control" group who received care at the Clinic, but not through the comprehensive care program, and a "non-attention" control group who could seek services elsewhere.

The study attempted to assess whether the utilization of hospital clinic facilities by mothers and their children increased for both immediate and preventive care, if there were any change in mother's general attitudes toward medicine and preventive care and if there were increased satisfaction experienced with doctor-patient contact in the Clinic.

The results were compared for the experimental and control groups and cross-tabulation of percentage distributions used to analyze the data.

The authors concluded that the institution of a comprehensive health care program did not change mother's general health attitudes and behavior, such as an increase in preventive health practices. However, increased satisfaction with health care was noted among mothers in the comprehensive program. The poor, then, the authors suggest, seem to prefer a primary care physician to whom they can go continually for health problems, rather than seeing any available doctor when they go to a clinic.

Andersen, R. and J. Kravits

　　　1971　　　"Disability days and physician contact for the two week period preceding the interview date by age, sex, race, residence, and family income." Preliminary Report No. 1 of research conducted under Contract Number HSM-110-70-392, NCHSRD. Chicago: Center for Health Administration Studies, University of Chicago.

The purpose of this report is to provide information on two-week use and disability days for a sample of the nation's population.

Data came from the 1971 CHAS-NORC national survey of health services utilization.

Information was reported on the mean physician visits in the past two weeks for those who had one or more disability days in that time period.

Also, a use-disability ratio was constructed by dividing the mean physician visits in two weeks for those who had one or more disability days by their mean disability days and multiplying by 100.

The use and use-disability rates were analyzed for different age, sex, race, residence and family income categories.

Cross-tabulation of rates was the mode of analysis employed.

For those with disability, the average number of disability days is greater for the poor at all ages. Among those with disability, poor urban blacks along with nonpoor urban whites are most likely to see a doctor. These findings, the authors suggest, may indicate that Medicaid, etc. are having some impact nationally. The poor and the rural populations have fewer visits per 100 disability days. Race *per se* does not appear to be related to this measure, however.

Andersen, R. and J. Newman

1973   "Societal and individual determinants of medical care utilization." *Milb. Mem. Fund Quart.* 51 (Winter): 95-124.

This paper suggests a comprehensive theoretical framework for the study of health services utilization.

Data are drawn from the Committee on the Costs of Medical Care (CCMC) study (1928-1931), CHAS (HIF)-NORC surveys (1953, 1958, 1964, 1971), NCHS data and other secondary data sources.

The authors point out that utilization may be considered in terms of the type (hospital, physician, drugs and medications, dentist, nursing home, etc.), purpose (primary, secondary, tertiary and custodial care) and unit of analysis (contact, volume, episodic care).

Some specific measures of utilization that appear in this article are mean physician visits per person per year, hospital admissions per 100 persons per year and the proportion with a dentist visit in the year.

The health delivery system is characterized by its resources and organization. Resources are described by their volume and distribution. Organization refers to the "access" ("means through which the patient gains entry to the medical care system and continues the treatment process") and structure of the system.

The population-at-risk is described by predisposing, enabling and need variables.

Data are presented in terms of cross-tabulations of percentages.

The framework presented emphasizes the importance of individual and societal determinants of utilization. It provides definitions of each of the outcome and process measures listed above and describes how they relate to one another conceptually.

It points out the demonstrated importance of the different individual determinants of physician, hospital and dentist utilization. Further, it introduces a framework for evaluating the intervention potential of model components in equalizing the distribution of health services — by their mutability, causation and interaction potential.

This article serves as the theoretical basis for the conceptualization of our access framework.

Andersen, R., et al.

1971   "The public's view of the crisis in medical care: an impetus for changing delivery systems?" *Econ. & Bus. Bulletin* 24 (Fall): 44-52.

This study is intended to report (1) the extent to which the public believes the system is in crisis; (2) the aspects of the system implicated as causing the crisis; and (3) consumer response to some of the proposals for changing the system.

Data came from the nationwide household survey of health care utilization and expenditures conducted by the Center for Health Administration Studies in 1971.

Public opinion was reported in terms of the percent who thought there was a crisis in health care in the United States today; the percent dissatisfied with the quality, cost, office waiting time, availability of medical care at night and on weekends, the ease and convenience of getting to a doctor, courtesy, information and coordination of medical care, respectively; and the percent favoring keeping, versus doing away with Medicare.

These opinions were analyzed by age, income and racial subgroups.

Percentage distributions were used to analyze the data.

Three-fourths of the sample agreed that there was a crisis in medical care. When aspects of the individual's own medical care were explored, the levels of dissatisfaction expressed were, in general, somewhat low. There were some aspects, especially cost and accessibility (gauged by waiting time, availability of care on night and weekends and ease and convenience of care), with which relatively high proportions of the sample were dissatisfied. Generally, people under 65 tend to be more dissatisfied than older people, nonwhites more dissatisfied than whites and the low-income more dissatisfied than the high-income. Some exceptions are the greater dissatisfaction by the younger, high-income groups with problems of access at night and on weekends and with getting information on care and coordinating it.

There was no consensus among this sample that universal government health insurance, such as through the extension of Medicare to those under 65, is the necessary solution to the health care crisis, however.

Andersen, R., et al.

1972   *Health Service Use: National Trends and Variations — 1953-1971.* Washington: National Center for Health Services Research and Development: U.S. Dept. HEW Publication No. (HSM) 73-3004.

The purpose of this study is to document trends in the public's use of health services in the United States and to consider major policy issues regarding the distribution of medical care according to age, income, race and residence.

Four parallel studies using household interviews were made of samples of the nation's families in 1953, 1958, 1964 and 1971.

The utilization indices were the source of regular care, percent seeing a physician during the survey year, mean number of physician visits per person-year, percent in hospital one or more days during survey year, hospital admissions per 100 person-years, in-hospital surgical procedures per 100 person-years, percent of women who saw doctor in first trimester of pregnancy, percent seeing a dentist during survey year, and mean number of dentist visits per person-year.

The characteristics of the population reported were age, sex, race, family income, residence and disability days. Characteristics of the delivery system, in terms of the Medicaid benefits available to the population in each state, were also reported.

Cross-tabulation of percentage distributions and rates are reported.

Findings from this report which support the view that the United States is attaining equalization of health care opportunity are as follows:

1) The gap between the percentage of low and high income people seeing a physician during the year narrowed considerably between 1963 and 1970. Most of the change was accounted for by an increase in the percentage of low-income children and young adults seeing the doctor.

2) The increase in the proportion of the population seeing a doctor between 1963 and 1970 among all age groups was greatest for the elderly.

3) Once they see a physician, low income people average *more* visits than those of higher income.

4) For those people seeing the doctor, the mean number of visits by non-whites is almost as great as the mean for whites and the mean number for central city residents exceeded the national average.

5) The lowest income people are almost twice as likely to be admitted to a hospital as those with the highest incomes in 1970 while in 1953 the admission rates were the same for all income groups.

(6) In 1963, the chances that pregnant women in the lowest income and education classes would see a doctor in the first trimester of pregnancy were less than one-half the chances for women with a college education and high family incomes. By 1970 most pregnant women, regardless of income or education, were seeing a doctor during the first trimester.

7) By 1970 the mean number of dental visits for persons seeing the dentist did not differ greatly according to income or race.

8) There was little difference in use of physicians in response to reported disability by blacks and whites.

Findings that contradict this picture of equalization include the following:

1) Low income people, nonwhites, and central city residents were considerably more likely than the rest of the population to have no regular source of care in 1970. Further, among people reporting a clinic as their regular source of care, the above groups are much less likely to see a particular doctor at the clinic.

2) A smaller proportion of the children living in central cities and rural areas see a doctor than is true for other children in the population.

Andersen, R., et al.

> 1973   *Expenditures for Personal Health Services: National Trends and Variations — 1953-1970.* Washington: Bureau of Health Services Research and Evaluation: U.S. Dept. HEW Publication No. (HRA) 74-3105.

The purposes of this study are (1) to indicate trends in personal health expenditures over time; (2) to examine the impact of financing programs, such as Medicaid and Medicare on such expenditures; and (3) to explore variations in expenditures in 1970 by selected social-demographic characteristics of the population.

The data are drawn from the 1964 and 1971 nationwide surveys of health services utilization conducted by the Center for Health Administration Studies, University of Chicago.

Mean expenditure for non-free personal health services per family, mean expenditures for all personal health services per family, aggregate family outlay for personal health services as a percent of family income, mean expenditure for non-free personal health services per person for all services and by type of service (hospital, physician, drugs, dentist, other), mean expenditures for personal health services per person for all services and by type of service, and mean expenditure and mean non-free expenditure per live birth served to reflect the volume of personal health services utilized.

The expenditure data were examined by age, sex, family income, poverty level, race, residence, and source of payment (Medicaid or Welfare, Medicare, voluntary insurance, out-of-pocket).

Simple cross-tabulation of percent distributions were used to analyze the data.

The authors conclude that the costs of medical care have been increasing, especially hospital services. Expenditures are greatest for the eldest age groups, whites and people living in the suburbs. When adjustments are made for family size, the poor and nonpoor have similar expenditures.

Aggregate family outlay for health services as a proportion of family income is higher for the poor than the nonpoor. While the overall proportion of family income spent for health services declined between 1958 and 1970, the proportion of low-income families continued to rise. Despite Medicaid, Medicare, etc., the poor continue to pay directly for a third of the services they received.

Voluntary insurance coverage pays the largest proportion of the hospital bill for all groups except the elderly, for whom Medicare is the chief payor, and the lowest income groups, for whom Medicaid and welfare pay. Direct consumer payment is still the major source of payment for physician services for all groups except the aged, who are covered by Medicare. Direct consumer payments also account for the major proportion of drug (84 percent) and dental (90 percent) expenditures. Medicaid and welfare appear to be making inroads into payment for maternity services and live births for low-income mothers.

The population groups that consistently have low expenditures for most types of services are (1) nonwhites; (2) low-income children living in rural areas; and (3) middle-income children and adults living in central cities.

Anderson, J.G. and D.E. Bartkus

    1972   "Choice of medical care: a behavioral model of health and illness behavior." Working Paper No. 63. Lafayette, Indiana: Institute for the Study of Social Change, Department of Sociology, Purdue University.

This study analyzes health and illness behavior in terms of a conceptual model that links sociodemographic characteristics to economic, ecological, need and social psychological variables and to a measure of health services utilization.

Data were collected from a random sample of students enrolled in a university health plan (N=946). Mailed questionnaires were used to collect the data.

The utilization index was created by dividing the number of visits to the university student health center by the total number of visits to all physicians and clinics during the same period of time.

The model included respondent's age, sex, marital status, attitudes toward the student health center and his perception of other students' appraisal of the student facility, his socio-economic status, the presence of additional insurance coverage, whether or not he had a regular family physician before coming to the university, whether he lived on campus, and his symptom sensitivity and "need for medical care" scores.

Path analysis was used to analyze the data.

The model suggested that social psychological factors such as symptom sensitivity and students' and friends' appraisal of the services provided affect the extent to which they seek outside medical care. While medical need and insurance coverage both directly affect the choice of health services, sociodemographic (age, sex, socio-economic status) and ecological (distance) factors appear largely to affect utilization indirectly through their effect on intervening social psychological variables.

Anderson, O.W.

    1972   *Health Care: Can There Be Equity?* New York: John Wiley and Sons.

This is a comparative study of health service systems in the United States, Sweden, and Great Britain.

Secondary data sources from each country, such as the Bureau of the Census, the Social Security Administration, American Hospital Association, National Center for Health Statistics and the Center for Health Administration Studies in the United States, the National Board of Health in Sweden and the Department of Health and Social Security in England and Wales provided the data reported in this study.

The author outlines the different elements of a health services system — indicators of units of facilities, use of facilities (hospitals, etc.), use of medical personnel (physicians, etc.), health level indicators and financial indicators.

He describes a model of a modern health service, how the elements relate to one another, and applies this model to explain the rise of services in the three countries, where the health care systems range from loosely to highly structured. Further, the author suggests an economic-political model common to all three countries but with widely varying philosophies of government intervention in and responsibility for health and welfare services. He shows what problems are inherent in any health system and what problems might be solved by government intervention.

Of special interest is that the author argues that some "indicators of equity," rather than general health indices, should be used to evaluate and compare different delivery systems. Such measurements might include who does and does not use the system, how and where different segments of the population enter the system and with what ailments, or the extent to which people experience difficulty or dissatisfaction with out-of-pocket costs, waiting time, etc., associated with gaining entry to the system.

Baggish, D.A. and C.P. Kimball

    1973   "The problem of transportation to medical facilities on an Indian reservation." *Med. Care* 11 (November-December): 501-508.

The purpose of this study is to determine the importance of transportation as a barrier to access to medical care for an Indian population.

Interviews with 171 outpatients at the Tuba City Public Health Service Hospital, Arizona, provided the data for this study.

Various questions were asked to elicit information about the difficulties experienced in trying to get to the Tuba City Hospital — family size, means of transportation, distance from hospital, distance from hogan to nearest main road, time of travel, cost of coming to hospital and reception to the idea of a bus.

Cross-tabulation of percentages and graphs were used to summarize the data.

No organized system of public transportation was found. Only 30 percent of the families interviewed owned vehicles. Most others came to the hospital by walking, hitchhiking or paying large fees to neighbors. Isolation, great distances, poor roads and long transit times were cited as problems. Seventy-four percent (74 percent) said they would use a bus, should it become available.

Beck, R.G.

1973   "Economic class and access to physician services under public medical care insurance." *Intl. J. Health Services* 3 (Summer): 341-355.

The purpose of this study is to analyze the impact of public medical care insurance on access to physician services.

Data are presented for the period 1963 through 1968 for a sample of families in the Province of Saskatchewan in Canada.

The measure of accessibility employed is the proportion of families of a given economic class who have *not* had medical services in a given year. The annual percentage of zero-users was computed for all services, general practitioner and specialist services, examinations, laboratory testing, home and emergency visits, hospital visits and major and minor surgery.

Graphs were used to portray the findings.

The evidence suggests that low-income classes have less contact with physicians than high-income classes. This disparity in accessibility is reduced, but not removed, as experience with public medical insurance increases. It is concluded that such insurance does result in increased *relative* accessibility to physicians for the low-income classes, though there may still be questions about what absolute level should be regarded as "non-equitable".

The authors use a "medical care iceberg" notion to conceptualize "access." The iceberg itself represents the set of medical needs that might be treated by a physician. The proportion of iceberg above water represents those needs which actually receive the attention of a physician. The greater the portion of the iceberg represented by the different income strata above water, the greater the "access" to care by those groups.

Becker, M.H., et al.

1972   "Motivations as predictors of health behavior."
Health Services Reports 87 (November): 852-862.

The purpose of this study is to hypothesize dimensions of motivations apt to affect adherence to medical regimens, develop and test measures of these dimensions and evaluate those variables as valid predictors of compliance.

The sample consisted of 125 female adults accompanying children being treated for otitis media in a comprehensive child care clinic at a large teaching hospital in 1971.

Compliance was measured by the administration of prescribed medications and keeping follow-up appointments. Long-run dependability was evaluated by the number of appointments kept divided by the number of appointments made during a twelve-month period.

Variables that were hypothesized to affect health motivation, and hence, compliance included perceptions of the physical threat of the illness, of control over health matters, general medical motivation and general concern about health.

Non-parametric measures of association were used to analyze the data.

A profile of the noncompliant mother is drawn from the data. She is little aroused by stimuli related to health matters. She sees her child as relatively healthy and likely to remain so. Consequently, she seems unlikely to want to undertake special activities for maintaining his health. The noncompliant mother is somewhat skeptical of a particular diagnosis and of the total medical care her child receives. The authors conclude that efforts to increase the health motivations of mothers toward compliance must be undertaken when such motivations are found to be inadequate.

Bellin, S.S. and H.J. Geiger

1972   "The impact of a neighborhood health center on patients' behavior and attitudes relating to health care: a study of a low-income housing project."
Med. Care 10 (May-June): 224-239.

This study reports the impact of the introduction of a neighborhood health center into a community on the population's utilization of and satisfaction with medical care.

Data were collected from two surveys of representative samples of residents of Columbia Point, a low-income, public housing community, of about 5,500 people in Dorchester, Massachusetts. The first survey was conducted in December, 1965, just prior to the introduction of the Tufts Health Center in the community, and the second two years later.

Health behavior was reported in terms of the percent who had asymptomatic general examinations, polio immunizations, and the percent who delayed in seeking care during the preceding six months.

Beliefs and sentiments relevant to health behavior were also reported. Beliefs regarding when a physician should be seen were reflected in knowledge of symptoms that warranted medical attention and belief in the value of asymptomatic checkups. Attitudes toward sources of ambulatory care were reflected in general evaluations of medical care and the health center, specific evaluation of what they did and did not like about the center, attitudes toward physicians at the center, and comparative evaluation of alternative sources of care.

The situational barriers to care studied were 1) the reasons cited for postponing needed medical care, 2) what barriers to the use of emergency services were reported, 3) the time spent in obtaining services, and 4) considerations of financial indebtedness incurred by poor health.

The data were reported in terms of cross-tabulation of percentage distributions.

The before-and-after data showed marked increases in the use of asymptomatic exams and poliomyelitis immunizations and a reduction in families who postponed needed medical care.

Recognition of symptoms of illness increased, as did the proportion who acknowledged the value of asymptomatic checkups. The proportion of residents who reported they were "very satisfied" with medical care increased from 56 to 81 percent. Ninety-six percent of the sample mentioned things they liked about the health center and only 37 percent things they did not like. Attitudes toward physicians improved. A majority of residents preferred the Health Center over its closest rival by a ratio of 2 to 1.

A marked decrease in the importance of the situational barriers to health care was also reported.

Berkanovic, E. and L.G. Reeder

> 1973   "Ethnic, economic and social psychological factors in the source of medical care." *Social Problems* 20 (Fall): 246-259.

The purpose of this study is to determine whether an "access" or a "cultural" explanation accounts better for the different patterns of health service use. If income alone predicted one's source of medical care, this would be evidence of an "access" explanation. If ethnicity predicted the source, there would be evidence of a "cultural" hypothesis.

A sample of 1,600 residents of Los Angeles County, California, were interviewed in the fall, 1970. There were 1,026 completed interviews.

The source of medical care an individual had received within the previous two months was broken down into two categories — private physician with own office and all others (outpatient department of a hospital, emergency room, clinic, etc.)

Characteristics of the population-at-risk reported included the income and ethnic group of the respondent and his orientation to the community and to the medical care system.

Cross-tabulation of percent distributions were used to analyze the data.

The authors conclude that there is a complex interaction between ethnicity and income in determining the source of medical care reported by the respondents. Neither the "access" nor "cultural" hypothesis alone can provide a full explanation. Ethnicity and income create different life experiences, which lead to differences in value preferences, including preferences for health care. Subcultures are of interest in that they create differences in social psychological orientations, which underlie behavior — behavior, here, being the choice of health care source.

Borkow, G.

1973   "Use of alternate facilities by consumers at the Providence Health Centers." *Inquiry* 10 (March): 54-58.

The purpose of this study is to analyze the factors that influence consumers' choices of alternative health facilities.

During a two-week period in May, 1972, a sample population of users of the Providence Health Centers, Inc. (PHC) — a low-income, consumer-controlled corporation operating out of ten storefront health centers in Providence, Rhode Island — were interviewed (n=195).

They were asked questions to determine their previous patterns of medical care seeking — "where did you last go for any kind of health care?"; "when did you go there?"; "what part of the week was this?"; and "how often do you use this facility?"

Certain demographic information — age, sex, race — were also collected, as was information on the proximity of the health center to a hospital.

A Kolmogorov-Smirnov test of statistical significance was performed on the data.

The author reports that PHC users were more apt to use alternative facilities, such as a hospital emergency room or outpatient department, when the center was in close proximity to such a facility.

Brooks, C.H.

1973   "Associations among distance, patient satisfaction, and utilization of two types of inner-city clinics." *Med. Care* 11 (September-October): 373-383.

The purpose of this study is to analyze the relationships among distance, patient satisfaction, and utilization of two types of inner-city clinics.

Data were collected from interviews of 160 respondents representing the users of "large-bureaucratic" clinics and 157 respondents who used "small-neighborhood" clinics in Detroit. All of the sample were black and 94 percent were female.

The number of times the respondent had attended the clinic and source of patient referral were reported. Consumer satisfaction with care was elicited by responses to questions about whether the patient thought the care received was "excellent, fair, or bad" and what could be done to improve service at the clinic.

Distance was reported as a straight-line distance between point of patient residence and point of clinic location. The type of clinic — large-bureaucratic or small-neighborhood — was based on the clinic's size and administrative structure.

Goodman-Kruskal's gamma was used as the test statistic.

The authors found that larger, bureaucratically administered clinics tend to increase the proportion of their user population as distance increases. Small neighborhood clinics, however, tend to draw their patients from within a half mile of them. Source of referral may explain these differences. As distance increases, a greater proportion of patients in large-bureaucratic clinics are formally referred to them, from elsewhere in the urban health bureaucracy. On the other hand, small-neighborhood clinics direct their services more to a neighborhood population. There appears to be no relationship between "frequency of attendance" and distance.

Even though about the same proportion of patients in both types of clinics express no criticism, patients in large-bureaucratic clinics tend to be more critical of professional staff and administrative procedure, while patients in small neighborhood clinics tend to focus their criticisms more on a clinic's physical appearance. The author advises that future research on consumer satisfaction should develop indexes that include not only the substantative nature and direction (positive or negative) of the comments, but the intensities with which they are expressed.

Bullough, B.

1972   "Poverty, ethnic identity and preventive health care." *J. Health Soc. Behav.* 13 (December): 347-359.

This study investigates the relationship between socio-economic status and the utilization of preventive health services.

A sample of 806 women from three poor neighborhoods in Los Angeles (one white, one black and one Mexican-American) were interviewed. All of the women had delivered a baby two to four months prior to the study.

The mothers' use of preventive services was reflected in their prenatal and postpartum care; their new baby's health; checkups, immunizations and dental care of their older children; and their own medical and dental care.

Information on the socio-economic status of respondents, their ethnic background and the level of alienation they felt — measured by feelings of powerlessness, hopelessness and social isolation — were reported.

Cross-tabulation of percentage distributions was used to report the findings.

The authors conclude that the lower a woman's socio-economic status, the less apt she is to seek preventive care for herself or her children. They suggest that alienation may act as an intervening variable to explain the underutilization of preventive care by the poor. Lack of money has a direct effect on the use of services, but the social psychological feelings of alienation, etc. that arise from being poor also have their indirect effect on the disadvantaged's use of preventive services.

Chen, M.K.

1973   "Access to health care: a preliminary model." Unpub. manuscript. National Center for Health Services Research and Development.

The purpose of this paper is to introduce some quantitative indicators of access.

The papers present hypothetical data only.

The author suggests that consumer satisfaction may be used as an external validator of some of the process indices he has developed.

Three indices he introduces are as follows:

(1) $C_1 = \sum_{j=1}^{3} V_j \sum_{i=1}^{n} W_i (I_i - R_i)$, where

I_i = ideal number of types of service, personnel or equipment,

R_i = actual number of types of service, personnel or equipment,

W_i = weight for the absolute difference between the ideal and actual number,

V_j = weight for given category (i.e., services, personnel, equipment).

(2) $C_2 = f(A,T,W,P)$, where

A = appointment waiting time in days
T = patient travel time
W = waiting room time
P = actual processing time, from contact to completion

(3) $I_x = \arcsin(10^k C_1/N)^{\frac{1}{2}} + \arcsin(10^r C_2/N)^{\frac{1}{2}}$, where

I_x = angular transformation of the two ratios C_1 and C_2 that is intended to make the two ratios additive and to stabilize their variances

k,r = single digit numbers

The author computes the indices using hypothetical data. In general, he urges some caution with respect to the use of the indices. The weights that reflect the relative importance of the availability of resources (C_1) or times (C_2) are, he points out, arbitrarily determined. He suggests that one might determine the optimal weighting factors, based on external criteria, such as patient satisfaction.

He summarizes the data requirements necessary to construct his indices and also provides a critique of the use-disability ratio.

Donabedian, A.

1972   "Models for organizing the delivery of personnel

health services and criteria for evaluating them.''
Milb. Mem. Fund Quart. 50 (October): 103-154.

This article provides a conceptual discussion of access.
It is not an empirical article *per se.*
The author represents methods of describing the delivery system —
staff composition, appointment procedure, departmentalization, etc. of
hospital, for example. He points out the temporal, spatial and socio-
organizational characteristics of access and describes ways in which the
organization of the payment and financing of care might be characterized in evaluating access.
He provides a summary of his view of the access concept that closely
parallels our own:

> The proof of access is use of service, not simply the presence of a
> facility. Access can, accordingly, be measured by the level of use
> in relation to 'need.' One should recognize, however, that clients
> and professionals evaluate 'need' differently. Further, one must
> distinguish two components in use of service: 'initiation' and 'con-
> tinuation.' This is because different factors influence each, though
> any one factor may influence both. It is hardly necessary to em-
> phasize that barriers to access are not only financial but also
> psychological, informational, social, organizational, spatial, tem-
> poral and so on.

Donabedian, A.

1973   *Aspects of Medical Care Administration.*
        Cambridge: Harvard University Press.

This book brings together a wealth of information required by a
medical care administrator for defining objectives, assessing the need
for services in an area, and deciding whether or not existing resources
are adequate.
The author discusses the values that are implicit in decisions regarding the delivery of medical services and how program objectives are
defined and competing ones resolved.
Considerable attention is devoted to the different ways that need
might be evaluated and descriptions of particular indexes of health and
morbidity and how information on them are collected.
Criteria and indicators for assessing the supply of resources, productivity and the relation of productivity to need and demand are considered.

Finally the methods for estimating the required amounts of services and resources, based on need and demand are discussed.

At one point, the author discusses "accessibility" itself as a concept. He argues that it implies something more than the mere "availability" of resource. It also, he says, "comprises those characteristics of the resource that facilitate or obstruct use by potential clients" (p. 419). Two kinds of accessibility are noted — socio-organizational and geographic. Socio-organizational attributes include all those attributes of the resources that either facilitate or hinder the efforts of the client to reach care — other than spatial attributes. For example, where physicians are concerned, factors influencing socio-organizational accessibility include such things as the sex of the provider, his specialization or fee scale and the race or income of the patient. Geographic accessibility refers to the _"friction_ of space" that is a function of the time and physical distance that must be traversed to receive care.

Elford, R.W., et al.

> 1972   "A study of house calls in the practices of general practitioners." _Med. Care_ 10 (September-October): 380-394.

The purpose of this study is to describe patterns in the use of house calls by general practitioners.

A non-random sample of fifteen (15) general practitioners, who were members of the Massachusetts Chapter of the American Academy of General Practice Collaborative Research Group and the Harvard Family Health Care Program provided the data.

House calls as a proportion of the total contacts between patients and physicians were studied.

Variables that were considered in describing the pattern of house calls were the patient's age, the type of care given, diagnostic category of the ailment, emotional-physical content of patient's complaint, discussion of other problems not related to the primary diagnosis and the time of day and week of the visit.

There were no formal tests of statistical significance applied.

The patient's dwelling was the site of the visit for a large proportion of the patients. Those visited at home were more apt to be elderly and were more likely to be patients with whom the doctor did not have a comprehensive and total relationship. Problems that were emotionally charged were disproportionately seen at home. House calls were made in greater amounts during non-standard office hours. The authors conclude that the house call is a way doctors have of improving communication and rapport and possibly improving compliance with prescribed diagnostic regimens.

Elliott, J.L.

1972 "Cultural barriers to the utilization of health services." *Inquiry* 9 (December): 28-35.

The purpose of this study is to assess the impact of selected cultural barriers on the use of needed medical services.

Data were collected from three communities in Nova Scotia. Two were rural communities — Tancook Islands and Upper Hammonds Plains — and one was more urban — Mulgrave Park. Each varied greatly in terms of its ethnic and sociocultural heritage.

The utilization index was the percent reporting one or more untreated symptoms.

Utilization was evaluated in terms of the residents' age, education, illness behaviors (immediate help source, self-treatment, home remedy usage), and evaluation of physicians (skepticism, satisfaction).

Cross-tabulation of percentage distributions were used to report the findings.

The cultural barriers (education, etc.) were more relevant in the two rural communities than in the urban one. Variables centering upon self-treatment tended to be more strongly associated with unattended symptoms in the rural communities, also. In the urban community and one of the rural communities, the percent reporting untreated symptoms was higher for those who reported high levels of dissatisfaction with physicians. In all communities, the higher the respondents' skepticism of physicians, the larger the percent of the population with untreated symptoms.

Enterline, P., et al.

1973 "The distribution of medical services before and after 'free' medical care — the Quebec experience." *New Eng. J. Med.* 289 (November 29): 1174-1178.

This article deals with the effects of the introduction of a compulsory, universal health insurance plan in Canada on individuals' utilization of health services.

The heads of 11,579 households in the Montreal Metropolitan Statistical Area were interviewed over a period of three years. Half of the individuals were interviewed in 1969-1970, prior to the introduction of Medicare — which covers all services of physicians in the home, office or hospital. The other half were interviewed in 1971-72, after the plan's inception.

Information on the use of services reported included the number of physician visits per person per year by site and the percent of symptoms for which a physician was seen. Selected measures of satisfaction described included the percent who thought the quality of care had improved, percent who delayed in seeking care and the percent of individuals who considered the care received at the last visit the best possible.

The family's income and the availability of care, in terms of travel, appointment and office waiting time were reported.

Tabulation of percentage distributions were used to summarize the findings.

Utilization of physician services by persons in lower income groups increased considerably after Medicare. The percentage of selected medical symptoms for which a doctor was seen increased from 62 percent to 73 percent, with all the increase being in the lower income groups. This shift resulted in increased satisfaction (measured by opinion of quality and level of delay) among the low-income groups and less satisfaction among the high-income. Appointment and office waiting time increased, with the largest increases occurring for the high-income consumers. This may explain their greater dissatisfaction with medical care after the introduction of Medicare.

Fabrega, H., Jr. and R.E. Roberts

1972a   "Ethnic differences in the outpatient use of a public charity hospital." *Amer. J. Public Health* 62 (July): 936-941.

The purpose of this study is to explicate the differences in patterns of hospital use by the three principal ethnic groups (Anglo-Americans, Mexican-Americans and blacks) who live in the area studied (southwestern United States).

The total number of persons who used the public charity hospital of a southwestern U.S. city during a three-month period in 1968 constituted the sample.

The age, sex and ethnicity of the users of the hospital facilities were reported.

Summations of the number of users by their age, sex, and racial categories constituted the data analysis.

Females were found to use the hospital more than males. Blacks used the facility more than the Anglo- or Mexican-Americans in the area. Anglos were underrepresented in the younger age groups who came to the hospital. The authors concluded that most patients who used the public charity hospital did so because they could not afford a private physician and/or there were few private physicians available in their neighborhood.

Fabrega, H., Jr. and R.E. Roberts

> 1972b   "Social-psychological correlates of physician use by economically disadvantaged Negro urban residents." *Med. Care* 10 (May-June): 215-223.

This study examines the role of social psychological variables in the utilization behavior of Negro-Americans.

A probability sample of low-income Negro-Americans drawn from two census tracts in Houston, Texas, was surveyed during the summer of 1968 regarding their socio-psychological attributes. One year later the same group was contacted and information on their use of medical services during the past year was requested.

Frequency of medical contacts was the utilization index reported.

Extremes on the utilization measure — those without medical care use and those with multiple contacts — were compared on the following correlates: anomie (using Srole scale); salience of health as an economic concern; perception of own health status compared to others; prevalence of psychosomatic symptoms (22-item Midtown Manhattan scale); attitudes toward doctors; and knowledge of existing health care in the area.

The t-test, sign and binominal tests of statistical significance were used to analyze the data.

The model introduced by the authors hypothesized that individuals who visited physicians frequently should regard health as more salient to them; perceive themselves in a poorer state of health; report more psychosomatic symptoms; manifest a lesser degree of anomie; demonstrate less negative attitudes toward physicians; and reflect more knowledge of the health care system. When age and sex were controlled, no comparisons produced a t-value large enough to reach the level required for significance.

Feldman, J.J.

1966   *The Dissemination of Health Information*. Chicago:
            Aldine Publishing Company.

The purpose of this study is to assess the influence that subjective factors such as the general public's beliefs and attitudes have on the use of medical services.

The data are drawn from a nationwide study conducted by HIF-NORC in 1955.

Utilization information was reported in terms of the number of doctor visits during the preceding year, the length of time since a doctor was last seen, regularity of obtaining a general physical exam, reasons for getting last exam, length of time since last exam, and the percent of public with symptoms who saw a doctor.

Consumer satisfaction with the medical and dental care received in the preceding year was also elicited.

These variables were analyzed in terms of the age, sex, education, occupational stratum, income, region and residence of the respondents. Further, data of their opinions toward medical care, knowledge about the importance of selected symptoms, sources of information, etc. were reported.

The data were portrayed in simple cross-tabulations.

The findings of the various use measures using the 1955 nationwide sample were reported. The percent of physicians and the public who say that one should see a doctor if specified symptoms appear, was much higher than the percent of persons reporting each symptom who say they actually saw a doctor. The percent of the public who reported they were satisfied with the medical (or dental) care they received in the last year was quite high. The level of health information varied by the socio-demographic characteristics of the respondents. Younger people, women, the better-educated, business professionals, higher income people, people from metropolitan areas or the East or Far West were apt to be the best informed.

Fink, R.

1973   "Analysis of utilization data." *Med. Care* 11
            (March-April Supplement): 109-116.

This paper deals with the measurement, analysis and explanation of utilization rates.

It is primarily a conceptual article, in that it points out the minimal data one should collect to evaluate utilization behavior.

Information the author deems should be continuously collected to evaluate utilization are as follows: 1) patient characteristics — age, sex, relationships to subscriber, family size, marital and family status, and type of insurance coverage; 2) provider characteristics — physician specialty and job function of physician providers; 3) context of medical service — data, place, and whether it was a scheduled or walk-in appointment; and 4) medical description of complaint — diagnosis, treatment and medical procedures employed.

Further, the author points up the importance of considering the episode of illness concept and new explanatory variables that might account for utilization rates — use of paramedical personnel, the state of disease at which help was sought, etc.

Foster, A., et al.

1973   "Use of health services in relation to the physical home environment of an Indian population." *Public Health Rep.* 88 (October): 715-720.

This study seeks to examine the impact of the home environment on health services utilization for an Indian population.

Data were collected from the health records of 224 females and 288 males on a reservation and paired with an environmental survey of their homes.

The average number of visits and reasons for preventive visits to a clinic were reported for the sample.

The utilization indices were considered by ailment for both males and females and in the context of the respondent's "average home rating."

Simple cross-tabulations were reported.

Females made more visits than males for preventive care and more visits for every category of ailment except accidents. Patients who visited the clinic for respiratory infections and infectious diseases and attended well-child clinics came from poor home environments. Women who came for pelvic exams were from better homes. Both males and females who did not seek preventive care also made fewer total visits to the clinic.

Fox, P.D.

1972   "Access to medical care for the poor: the federal perspective." *Med. Care* 10 (May-June): 272-277.

This article is a conceptual discussion of aspects of access.
It does not present data as such.
The author discusses utilization as a kind of outcome indicator of
access.

He points up two main barriers to access — the supply and organization of medical resources in the system and the financial resources of the
population-at-risk — and the value of considering these in the context of
peoples' utilization of health services, to evaluate their "access" to
care.

Freeborn, D.K. and M.R. Greenlick

1973   "Evaluations of the performance of ambulatory care
            systems: research requirements and opportunities."
            Med. Care 11 (March-April Supplement): 68-75.

The purpose of this article is to specify the dimensions of utilization,
satisfaction and "appropriateness" of access that it is relevant to consider in evaluating the performance of an ambulatory care system.
The article is a conceptual, rather than an empirical one.
Utilization, in terms of the continuity of care, can be evaluated by the
extent to which services are person-centered or directed toward physical and psychosocial human needs; integrated and comprehensive; available through a central source; and coordinated as the patient moves
through the system. The general types of information needed to assess
continuity are as follows:

1) number of patients who have and use a central coordinated source
   of care and/or a primary physician;
2) frequency and appropriateness of referrals and consultations;
3) degree of compliance, particularly with respect to high-risk patients; and
4) degree of follow-up of abnormal findings.

Indices of patient satisfaction can be based on measurements of his
perceptions of the accessibility of services and the quality of care; the
process of care and the nature of interpersonal relationships involved;
and the system arrangements.
Satisfaction with accessibility and quality may be indicated by patients' attitudes and knowledge regarding 1) the extent to which services
are available at the time and place needed; and 2) the outcome of illness
— whether the patient perceived a change in his condition as a result of
care.

Satisfaction with the process of care is reflected in the following dimensions:

1) the extent to which patients value the availability of a primary care physician or central source of care;
2) the perception of the physician's and other personnel's interest and concern;
3) the degree of trust and confidence in the physician;
4) the degree of understanding of the condition or diagnosis; and
5) the extent to which there is difficulty understanding the physician's instructions.

The level of satisfaction with system arrangements may be gauged by attitudes toward 1) physical surroundings and facilities; 2) patient flow that includes the appointment system, waiting and processing time, helpfulness of personnel and the mechanisms used for solving complaints; and 3) the scope and nature of the benefits and services offered.

In addition to the attitudinal measures of satisfaction, there are several behavioral observations that can be made, also:

1) extent of medical care outside the system;
2) proportion of subscribers who leave the program and choose other health plans;
3) number and type of complaints received by the system;
4) broken appointments and cancellation rates;
5) rates of compliance with prescribed regimens; and
6) proportion of patients who change physicians, assuming there is a choice within the system.

With respect to "accessibility" *per se,* the authors argue that there are several criteria against which it can be measured. Ideally, individuals should have access to the system at the time and place needed, through a well-defined and known point of entry. A comprehensive range of personnel, facilities, and services that are known and convenient to the population should be available. In addition, there should be access and use that is proportional and appropriate to need. Specific information needed to evaluate access is as follows:

1) definition of the population to be served or eligible for care, and its social and demographic characteristics; these data are essential to identify the population-at-risk and to provide denominators for the utilization indices;
2) social and demographic characteristics, by selected morbidity, mortality, and disability rates, and by utilization patterns; these data aid in evaluating the relationship between need and use;

3) population groups with identifiable diseases not yet diagnosed; or diagnosed but not yet under treatment; such data assist in identifying unmet need; and
4) utilization patterns by time, place, type of service, type of provider, by presenting and associated morbidity and symptoms, and by episodes and procedure; this information helps describe the pattern of the process of care-seeking.

Freidman, B., et al.

1973   "The influence of medical and private health insurance on the early diagnosis of breast cancer." *Med. Care* 11 (November-December): 485-490.

The purpose of this study is to analyze the impact of insurance coverage on the stage of cancer at which care is sought.

Data for breast cancers first treated in 1970 were provided by the Massachusetts Tumor Registry.

The stage of cancer at which care was first sought served as the dependent variable.

The predictor variables analyzed were age, marital status, histology (American Cancer Society cases), insurance, previous tumor history and a series of variables on the housing situation in the respondent's area of residence (as proxy for income).

A single-equation multiple regression technique was used to analyze the data.

The results do not support the view that eliminating the direct expense to medical care consumers through the insurance is a meaningful stimulus to the early diagnosis of cancer.

Gibson, G.

1973   "Evaluative criteria for emergency ambulance systems." *Soc. Sci. Med.* 7 (June): 425-454.

This study attempts to construct a number of input, process and dispositional criteria to evaluate the provision of ambulance services in a community.

The study draws on over 50 evaluative surveys of emergency ambulance services in the United States and from a recent survey of emergency medical care in Chicago reported in the book, *Emergency Medical Services in the Chicago Area,* Chicago: Center for Health Administration Studies, University of Chicago, 1970.

Ambulance utilization rates reported are as follows: Fire Department, Police Department, total municipal, total private and total number of ambulance runs per 1,000 population; runs per year per Fire Department, Police Department, municipal and private ambulance; and proportion of "no service" runs, for Fire Department, Police Department, municipal and private ambulances.

Characteristics of ambulance users — age, sex, race and Census tract of residence — and of the delivery system — Fire Department, Police Department, total municipal, total private and total municipal and private ambulances per 100,000 population are also reported.

The author introduces a typology for ambulance program evaluation that is a kind of use-need discrepancy index:

		Clinically determined need for ambulance services	
		HIGH	LOW
Actual receipt	YES	A	B
of ambulance			
services	NO	C	D

He points out that the ambulance availability rates and ambulance utilization rates described earlier refer to what he would call "input" criteria. He argues that evaluative surveys of ambulance service must go beyond these measures to some kind of "process" and "dispositional" criteria.

The author goes on to describe three process criteria: (1) incidence and items of first aid rendered by ambulance personnel; (2) emergency rating and extent of injuries of ambulance cases; and (3) total response time from initial call to ambulance arrival at hospital.

With respect to the second criterion, he constructs an ambulance specifity index and an index of appropriate utilization based on his use-need typology. The ambulance specificity index, $D/B+D$, is the proportion of all patients not needing ambulance service who did not receive it. The index of appropriate utilization, $A/A+B$, is the percent of those who got care that needed it.

Some dispositional criteria the author suggests might be employed to evaluate ambulance services in an area are: (1) the proportion of ambulance cases taken to hospitals rated as providing comprehensive emergency treatment; (2) proportion of ambulance cases taken to hospitals with 400 or more beds; and (3) proportion of ambulance cases taken to hospitals with at least one approved residency or intern program.

Further, Gibson discusses the problem of unmet need. Some criteria he proposes to evaluate this are (1) proportion of all hospital emergency department patients who receive ambulance services; and (2) the proportion of hospital emergency department patients in need of ambulance service who received it.

The second index is called an ambulance sensitivity index and, based on the typology, is defined as A/B+C. Need is evaluated by physicians in terms of whether it is emergent, urgent, non-urgent or a scheduled procedure.

Gibson concludes with data from Chicago that show the ambulance sensitivity index to be low, 19 percent. The ambulance specificity index, however, is 84 percent. "Chicago ambulances can claim little abuse of its service (people who don't need them don't use them) but at the price of substantial unmet need."

Gibson, G., et al.

1970   *Emergency Medical Services in the Chicago Area.*
         Chicago: Center for Health Administration Studies,
         University of Chicago.

The purpose of this study is to describe and evaluate the organization and availability of emergency medical services in the City of Chicago.

A variety of data collection mechanisms were used — literature review, compilation of standards, mail questionnaires to ambulance companies and public officials, on-site surveys, hospital log book abstracts and patient interviews.

Data on the utilization of ambulance and emergency services and the characteristics of the users and the system itself are reported.

The data are presented as cross-tabulated percentages and rates.

The authors note the sharp increase in the use of the emergency room for non-urgent conditions since the early 1950's. The public and private ambulance systems in Chicago and suburban Cook County are described and evaluated. The availability of vehicles, in both private and municipal sectors in Chicago, does not compare favorably with other major U.S. cities. Recommendations with respect to the focus of responsibility for ambulance service among the Fire Department, Police and private sectors in Chicago are summarized.

Communications between the public ambulance dispatch offices and between ambulances and hospital emergency departments are described. Recommendations are made for more centralized dispatching and control.

Using the various minimum standards suggested by professional medical bodies, the emergency room facilities of Chicago hospitals are found to compare favorably with other metropolitan areas and to be in substantial compliance with relevant standards.

Several chapters are devoted to describing the characteristics of patients treated at hospital emergency rooms in Cook County. The financial characteristics of hospital emergency departments are described and a commentary on the role of emergency services within the wider context of the health care system presented. An extensive bibliography on emergency medical care is found at the conclusion of the report.

Gish, O.

1973   "Resource allocation, equality of access, and health." *Intl. J. Health Services* 3 (Summer): 399-412.

Based on the experience of Tanzania, this paper relates resource allocation in the health sector to the utilization of services by urban and rural populations.

Secondary analyses of official sources of data on health expenditures and output in Tanzania are reported.

Utilization is reflected in the number of inpatients per bed and the total outpatients by type of facility.

Financial input is represented by the total amounts of capital invested in the different facilities.

Cross-tabulation of rates are used to report the data.

The author suggests that "inequality of access" is reflected in the unequal amounts of capital expenditures for health in urban and rural areas. Because of the difficulty of measuring health outputs that are a direct result of these financial inputs, volume of services is offered by the authors as the "best available indicator of health output." According to the data presented here, there are more financial inputs provided to urban health care centers and, subsequently, substantially larger amounts of "health outputs" (i.e., utilization).

The authors conclude that building larger hospitals in underserved areas is not the answer to the problem. The major obstacles to change are not shortages of resources or technologic ignorance, but social systems that do not place a high value upon the health care needs of rural peasants.

Gordon, D.W.

1973   "Post-hospital discharge: patient care and utiliza-
          tion of services and facilities." *Inquiry* 10 (De-
          cember): 41-48.

The purpose of this study is to determine the disposition and status of
a representative sample of patients discharged from the New York
Hospital.

The sample was comprised of 358 respondents to a questionnaire
survey of 545 randomly selected patients discharged from six services of
the New York Hospital.

The disposition and type of care received by these respondents after
their discharge was reported.

Information on the patients' primary diagnoses was also collected.

Cross-tabulation of percentage distributions were used to report the
findings.

During the three-month post-discharge period, 91.8 percent of the
respondents returned home. The remaining 8.2 percent spent some time
in a hospital or extended care facility during this three-month period.
Eighty-two percent of these patients had primary diagnoses involving
malignant neoplasms, diseases of the circulatory system, and diseases of
the nerve and sense organs. Approximately seven percent (7%) of the
respondents were not ambulatory following their discharge and received
some sort of assistance in their family setting. Fifteen percent (15%)
were not ambulatory, but did not report receiving assistance during their
convalescence. Among those who required assistance 61.3 percent had
the following primary diagnoses: diseases of the circulatory system (25.8
percent); diseases of the nerve and sense organs (19.4 percent); malignant neoplasms (16.1 percent). The author argues that some of these
patients would not require placement in an extended care facility, but
could receive care in a low-cost minimal care facility within the hospital
for a brief period to avoid some of the problems of post-discharge
discontinuity.

Graf, W.S., et al.

1973   "A community program for emergency cardiac care:
          a three year coronary ambulance paramedic evalua-
          tion." *JAMA* 226 (October 8): 150-160.

This paper evaluates the effectiveness of a Coronary
Ambulance/Paramedic Program in the City of Los Angeles.

The number of individuals who required emergency ambulance service for cardiac care during each of the three years of the study served as the sample. They came from the 700,000 residents of varying socioeconomic status and ethnic groups, who lived in a ten-mile area of Los Angeles.

The number of individuals using the Coronary Care Unit (CCU) served as the utilization index.

A number of criteria were used to evaluate this program — which provided pre-hospitalization coronary care through ambulances that used specially-trained CCU nurses and paramedics. Seriously ill-patients who may have died on the way to the hospital, survived because of the attention they received in route. Publicity about the CCU resulted in an increase in calls for the ambulance in cardiac emergencies. Alerting of the hospital staffs about the patient's condition via radios in route permitted the staff to prepare more effectively for his arrival. The community seemed to readily accept the new role of the CCU paramedics.

Green, J. and J. Scharff

1971 "Use of medical services under Medicare." *Soc. Sec. Bull.* 34 (March): 3-16.

This article presents findings for 1967 from the Current Medicare Survey (CMS) on the use of medical services under the program and their relation to selected economic and social characteristics of the aged.

The Current Medicare Survey sample consists of about 4,500 persons selected from a five-percent statistical sample of persons enrolled in the supplementary medical insurance program, used in the basic Medicare data system.

Information is reported on the total and average number of physicians' visits (ambulatory and hospital) and charges under the supplementary medical insurance (SMI) program, and use and charges for prescription drugs.

This utilization and cost information are examined for different characteristics of the population covered under SMI: age, sex, race, education, health limitations, marital status, living arrangement, household size, work status, family income, private health insurance coverage, welfare status, region and residence.

Persons using services at higher rates tend to be older, confined to the bed or house, and to reside in urban areas. Typically they are nonworkers, are alone in the household, and have received some welfare services in the year. Persons utilizing medical services at lower rates tend to be relatively younger, have no health limitation, be rural residents, and are more likely to be employed.

In general, the characteristics of persons who met the $50 deductibles are similar to those of persons who are likely to use medical services in the first place.

To pay deductible and co-insurance amounts, persons frequently rely on themselves, a private health insurance plan, and welfare funds as primary sources of payment.

About four-fifths of all enrollees acquired prescription drugs. Older persons, those with some health limitations, and persons not working were more likely to use prescription drugs.

Greenlick, M.R., et al.

1973   "Determinants of medical care utilization: the role of the telephone in total medical care." *Med. Care* 11 (March-April): 121-134.

The purposes of this study are to report data depicting various aspects of the telephone utilization of a prepaid group practice plan membership and to examine physicians' behavior in response to calls from patients.

Data came from a five percent sample of Kaiser Plan enrollees in 1969 (n=5,191). Clinic records were examined to collect the data.

The number, type and disposition of the call was reported.

Calls were examined in terms of the age, sex and family size of the caller, his presenting symptom and morbidity, whether the call was for an initial or continuing episode, and whether the doctor responding was the caller's regular or temporary attending physician.

Cross-tabulation of percentage distributions and a Chi-square test of significance were performed on the data.

Telephone calls represented a significant proportion of the total medical care of the sample studied. The differences by age, sex and family size were quite small. About 50 percent of all phone calls were concerning symptoms and approximately 40 percent concerned laboratory results or prescriptions.

The study hypothesized that the relative probability of a patient being told to come to the clinic after discussing a symptom would vary inversely with the certainty of the physician in his diagnosis and directly with the seriousness of the disease as perceived by the physician. The inferences from the data support this hypothesis. It is difficult to predict from the data, given the wide individual variation among physicians, when a physician would only discuss the symptom, give a prescription, or request a patient to come for a visit, however.

Hackett, T.P., et al.

1973   "Patient delay in cancer." *New Eng. J. Med.* 289 (July 5): 14-20.

This study describes some of the reasons people might delay in seeing a doctor, once symptoms of cancer are perceived.

The tumor registry questionnaire at Massachusetts General Hospital for patients who registered between 1963 and 1970 constituted the data source for this study (n=563).

Delay was defined as the time from the patient's first awareness of symptom or sign to the first consultation with a physician (0-1 week, 2-4 weeks, 1-3 months, 7-12 months, more than a year).

Information collected on the patients included why they first saw a doctor — pain, incapacity, physical exam, worry, advice of friend; what they called the condition — tumor or cancer; site of the cancer; family history of cancer; self-ratings of procrastination in seeing doctors; worrying; and the social class of the respondent.

The findings showed that detection of cancer through routine physician examinations insured the least delay. Worry about the condition reduced delay time more than pain, incapacity, or other factors. Patients of higher social class sought help significantly sooner than the less privileged. Those who openly referred to their condition as cancer delayed less than those who used the term, "tumor." Delay appeared to be a conscious and deliberate act rather than a failure to perceive the neoplasm and its consequences.

Hassinger, E.W. and J.C. Belcher

1973   "Patterns of access to health services in rural areas." Unpub. manuscript. Columbia, Missouri: Department of Rural Sociology, University of Missouri.

The purpose of this paper is to describe the characteristics of rural society and the health delivery organization in rural areas in an effort to explain the patterns of access to medical care that exist for the rural population.

This paper is not empirical *per se,* but draws on National Center for Health Statistics data and other studies to describe the rural population's "access" to medical care.

The authors cite data on hospital, physician and dentist use in rural areas. Statistics on hospital discharges from short-stay general hospitals, mean number of physician visits, the site of the visit, the types of providers seen, the preventive service use rate, the pattern of physician referrals and mean dental visits served as the utilization indices.

Utilization was examined in terms of the age, education, race, attitudes toward medicine, income, insurance coverage, organization of services, supply of medical personnel and distance from care of the rural population.

The paper shows that the rural population is apt to be younger, poorly educated and have lower incomes and less insurance coverage than the urban population. The rural population averages slightly more hospital use than city people. Rural residents consistently report fewer physician visits, are less apt to see physicians at clinics, such as the ones available to low-income city residents, more often see general practitioners than specialists, have lower preventive service use rates and are not necessarily referred to specialists by their family doctors, but must seek out such practitioners themselves. Rural people also average fewer dentist visits annually.

The authors conclude that these differences are not due to the attitudes and medical beliefs of the rural population themselves, but to the organizational problems associated with distance, the undersupply of medical manpower and the lack of integrated referral networks in the rural areas.

Hassinger, E.W. and D.J. Hobbs

> 1972   *Health Service Patterns in Rural and Urban Areas: A Test Between Availability and Use.* Research Bulletin 987. Columbia, Missouri: Agricultural Experiment Station, College of Agriculture, University of Missouri.

This study's expressed objective is "to examine the difference in level and pattern of use of health services within the context of availability of services in rural and urban communities."

The data were collected from surveys done in four rural and one urban (Springfield) community in Missouri during 1967. Springfield, in contrast to the rural communities, offered a full-range of medical specialization and complex health facilities.

Level of use was gauged by the number of physician visits per individual per year, percent using hospital during the year and percent using marginal practitioners, such as chiropractors. The variables representing pattern of use were the number of different doctors used, use of specialists versus general practitioners, percent having family doctors and source of referrals.

Use was examined for each of the five communities, for the four rural communities compared to the urban one, and by the age, education and income of the female household heads and the age of individuals in household.

Cross-tabulation of percentage distributions were used to analyze the data.

In contrast to an hypothesized relationship, level and pattern of use among the four rural communities were similar and differences between rural communities and the urban community were relatively small. Urban people at each age level were more likely to make use of physicians' services during the year and to report hospital experience, but the differences were very small. Urban people tended to use chiropractors more often, simply because such practitioners were more available to them.

Families in the urban community tended to use more different doctors than rural families, but this difference was reduced when individuals were considered. Urban families were much more likely to use specialists — once again, because they were more available to them. There was little difference in the rural and urban samples in the proportions who reported having a family doctor. Similarly, professional and lay referral patterns were parallel in the rural and urban populations.

Greater internal differentiation in the use of medical services — such as by income — was, in contrast to one of the hypotheses of the study, not found to be greater in the urban community.

The authors conclude that because of the similarity or urban and rural use patterns, perhaps less emphasis should be placed on the expensive relocation of health centers to serve rural populations.

Also, see article by authors, entitled "The relation of community context to utilization of health services in a rural area," *Med. Care* 11 (November-December): 509-522.

Hassinger, E.W. and R.L. McNamara

1973   *Changes in Health Behavior and Opinions among*

*Open-Country Families in Two Missouri Counties
1955-56 and 1968.* Research Bulletin 994. Columbia,
Missouri: Agricultural Experiment Station, College
of Agriculture, University of Missouri.

This study analyzes changes in health behavior and opinions of a rural
population that occurred over the decade 1955-56 to 1968, in which
substantial changes in the focus of public policy of the problems of rural
areas occurred.

Baseline surveys of rural populations in two counties in Missouri,
Harrison and Laclede Counties, were undertaken in 1955-56. A fol-
lowup survey in the same counties was conducted in 1968. The family
was the unit of analysis in each survey.

The following indicators of health behavior and opinions were
analyzed: utilization of health services, method of paying for services,
health maintenance, opinions about physicians, family doctor relationship and selected health practices.

Utilization was examined for hospital, physician and dentist services.
The percent of survey families with any hospitalization and the number
of hospital days, the percent families with any physician visits and the
number of visits, and the percent of families with any dentist visits
constituted the utilization indices.

The method of payment for health services was described by the
percent of families with health insurance coverage and response to
hypothetical situation of how family would pay for a medical bill of $100,
$500, $1,000, or $5,000.

Health maintenance responses were elicited by questions regarding
how often one should see a doctor and dentist, and whether the family
actually does have routine physical and dental examinations.

Opinions about physicians were reflected in questions about respondents' general faith in physicians and whether they flet that they needed
care but did not receive it for any reason.

The relationship to a family doctor was determined by the percent of
families who reported having a family physician, the percent who talk
over problems other than health problems with their family doctor and,
percent agreeing with more generalized statements about desired level
of interaction with physician.

Other health practices referred to the possession of a fever thermometer and a doctor book and related health behavior, such as dieting and the
use of vitamins.

Each of the dimensions of health opinions and behavior cited above
were examined for the age and education of the household head and the

level of living, based on income and related economic indexes. The authors hypothesized that changes in the two counties over the period between the two surveys is apt to be due to 1) the general rise in level of living in rural areas; 2) the trend toward secularization; and 3) the "leveling" of intra-rural differences between the counties.

A Chi-square test of significance was performed on the data.

Changes on the indices of use of health services over time were not dramatic. The authors argue that until major changes in the delivery system occur, such changes are not likely to be forthcoming. The volume of use in each county was quite similar.

The level of insurance coverage increased over time, especially for those with high level of living scores. The volume of increase was similar in the two counties.

Secularization was predicted to lead to an increase in the expressed value and seeking of health maintenance practices. The data from both Harrison and Laclede Counties bore out this hypothesis.

Expected deterioration in "regard for physicians" and perception of greater unmet medical needs due to secularization was not borne out.

The family doctor relationship was also fully maintained and increased in significance in Harrison County. At the same time, the personal quality of the relationship diminished.

The possession of a fever thermometer and use of vitamins increased, but possession of doctor book and dieting showed little change.

Hassinger, E.W., et al.

1970   *Extent, Type, and Pattern of Use of Medical Services in a Rural Ozark Area.* Research Bulletin 965. Columbia, Missouri: Agricultural Experiment Station, College of Agriculture, University of Missouri.

The objective of this study is to explore how the internal structures of communities (age, socio-economic status, etc.) relate to the extent, type and pattern of health service used in a rural area.

Data were collected from a survey of four rural communities in South Central Missouri during the summer of 1967.

The extent or volume of use was gauged by the number of doctors and the number of physician visits by families and individuals and the percent of families and individuals hospitalized and their length of hospital stay.

The type of practitioners used were analyzed according to whether they were general practitioners or specialists and the percent of families and individuals who used osteopaths and chiropractors.

The pattern of use was analyzed in terms of whether or not families had a family physician and the patterns of referral to specialists.

These different dimensions of use were analyzed by the age and education of the female head of the household and family income.

Cross-tabulation of percentage distributions were used to analyze the data.

For most families and individuals, use was confined to one or two doctors during the survey year. The average number of physician visits and amount of hospitalization per individual compares closely to National Center for Health Statistics data on such indices by age, income, etc. Young families were equally likely to make some use of doctors, regardless of income. In the older age categories, however, the use of services was typically greater for higher income families.

Use of full-time specialists increased with age of family and also with family income. The use of osteopaths was indistinguishable from that of general practitioners in terms of the characteristics of patients who see them. Chiropractors, however, were more often seen for particular ailments.

Most families reported a family doctor relationship, regardless of age, education and income differences. Existence of a family doctor did not preclude the widespread self-initiated use of other local general practitioners and specialists, however.

Hastings, J.E.F., et al.

1973   "Prepaid group practice in Sault Ste. Marie, Ontario. Part I. Analysis of utilization records." *Med. Care* 11 (March-April): 91-103.

The purpose of this study was to compare the utilization experience of a prepaid group practice plan membership with families who got care from independent practitioners, using medical records.

Data from the analysis of the medical records of Canadian steel workers — some of whom were enrolled in a Group Health Association (GHA) prepaid group practice plan and the others who received care from independent practitioners through an indemnity plan (IIP) — supplied the data. The study took place during the period July 1, 1967 through June 30, 1968.

Both hospital and physician utilization data were reported. Hospital utilization rates (discharges, length of stay, days per 1000 person-years), the amount and type of surgery, hospital readmission rates, percent who saw physician, number of visits, type of service received, provider and the number of radiologic and laboratory services used comprised the utilization indices.

These utilization rates were compared for the GHA and other union members.

Cross-tabulation of distributions and rates constituted the data analysis.

GHA plan members were found to: 1) spend 24 percent less time in the hospital, mainly due to lower admission rates; 2) have fewer surgical operations; 3) have lower rates of hospital readmission; 4) were more likely to have seen a physician at least once in the previous 12 months; 5) more likely to receive immunizations and check-up; 6) more likely to be attended by "appropriate" specialists; and 7) to undergo more radiologic and laboratory investigations, especially on an outpatient basis.

Hetherington, R.W. and C.E. Hopkins

1969   "Symptom sensitivity: its social and cultural correlates." *Health Services Research* 4 (Spring): 63-75.

The purpose of this study is to examine the impact of an individual's perception of the severity of his symptoms on his orientation to action or inaction in consulting a doctor.

A sample of 238 subscribers to three health insurance plans in Los Angeles provided the data.

Respondents were given a list of symptoms and asked to check those for which they thought it necessary to consult a physician. Ten (10) physicians were also asked to rate the symptoms. Each individual's score was compared with the physicians' scores. In this manner, respondents were divided into three groups: 1) symptom-insensitive — individuals who failed to check symptoms physicians rated as serious; 2) symptom-sensitive — those who agreed with physicians; and 3) symptom-hypersensitive — those checking symptoms the physician thought trivial.

Information was collected on the demographic characteristics — age, sex and marital status; cultural characteristics — cultural and ethnic groups; socio-economic characteristics — social class and social status within the community — of the three groups.

Cross-tabulation of percentage distributions were used to analyze the data.

Middle-aged respondents were significantly hypersensitive, particularly female, the formerly married and those in high occupational categories. Low prestige ethnic background was related to symptom insensitivity for those who were upwardly mobile, as compared to their fathers. Low income was related to symptom insensitivity for those with high-status ethnic and religious backgrounds and for those who were downwardly mobile or non-mobile occupationally.

Hillman, B. and E. Charney

> 1972   "A neighborhood health center: what the patients
>   know and think of its operation." *Med. Care* 10
>   (July-August): 336-344.

This study was undertaken to evaluate the effectiveness of a neighborhood health center, particularly in terms of the patients' knowledge of and satisfaction with the facility.

Data were collected from open-ended interviews with one adult member of families selected at random from families registered with the Rochester, New York, Neighborhood Health Center.

Information was collected on the regular sources of health care for the family, the patients' perception of the nature and hours of operation of the facility and their satisfaction or dissatisfaction with the facility.

The effect of the center was portrayed in cross-tabulations of responses to the preceding questions.

The study demonstrated that the comprehensive care offered by the health center was accepted enthusiastically by a majority of the neighborhood residents. Patients generally liked the doctors, nurses and "health assistants" at the Center, and felt they were receiving good medical care. Fourteen of the patients interviewed reported using outside care sources occasionally. Thus, the Center may not meet all the patients' primary care demands. Some patients expressed the concern that the residents should exercise some type of community control over the Center.

Hulka, B.S., et al.

> 1971   "Satisfaction with medical care in a low-income
>   population." *J. Chronic Dis.* 24 (November):
>   661-673.

The purpose of this study is to analyze the satisfaction of a low-income population with medical care.

Data were collected from a household survey conducted in the fall of 1969 among 254 low-income adult respondents in Raleigh, North Carolina.

A satisfaction questionnaire was constructed in accordance with Thurstone's Equal Appearing Interval Technique. Three elements of attitudes toward physicians were tapped: professional competence, personal qualities and cost/convenience. Respondents received a total score, as well as a score reflecting their level of satisfaction or dissatisfaction with each content area.

The satisfaction scores were analyzed in relation to family size, education, occupation, regular source of care, insurance coverage, recent doctor visit or not and race.

Correlation analysis, t-tests and Chi-square tests of significance were used to analyze the data.

The distribution of scores were found to be significantly more favorable on personal qualities (mean value of 65.2) as compared to cost/convenience (mean 49.1). Scores on professional competence had an intermediate distribution (mean 58.5). These means were statistically different from each other.

Increased satisfaction with professional competence was associated with higher educational and occupational levels. Increased family size resulted in decreased satisfaction with costs and convenience. Having hospital insurance, a regular doctor and a recent doctor visit were correlated with higher total satisfaction scores.

Hulka, B.S., et al.

1972   "Determinants of physician utilization: approach to a service-oriented classification of symptoms." *Med. Care* 10 (July-August): 300-304.

The purpose of this study is to explain utilization behavior in a low-income population.

A random probability sample of residents of low-income census tracts in Raleigh, North Carolina, in fall, 1969, provided the data. In total, 495 residents in 160 households were interviewed.

The utilization index was doctor visits versus no doctor visits made during the four weeks prior to the interview.

Correlates examined included age, sex, race, number of symptom-complexes per person, worry caused by illness, seriousness, as respondent saw it of complaint, perceived doctor's ability to relieve complaint, duration of complaint, number of activity-loss days, and number of bed-loss days.

Stepwise regression and Chi-square test of significance were the modes of analysis used.

The findings showed that 117 out of 140 doctor visits were symptom-oriented. Seriousness of complaint, bed-loss days, perceived doctor's ability to relieve the complaint, and race were entered in stepwise regression, in that order, as the predictors that discriminated between those who had contacted a doctor and those who had not.

Hurtado, A.V., et al.

    1972   "The utilization and cost of home care and extended care facility services in a comprehensive, prepaid group practice program." *Med. Care* 10 (January-February): 8-16.

This article reports on a project designed to provide home care and extended care facility services presently available under Medicare to a population of more than 100,000 people under 65 years of age in a comprehensive, prepaid group practice program.

Records of the membership of the Kaiser Foundation Health Plan provided the data.

Utilization information was collected in terms of acute hospital and extended care facility utilization (number of discharges, number of days, average length of stay, discharges per 1,000 members, days per 1,000 members), home care utilization (admissions, days, average stay, admissions per 100,000 hospitalized, days per 100,000 hospitalized), and total home care visits and procedures for type of visit by type of procedure.

These use rates were analyzed for different age groups.

Simple cross-tabulation of percentage distributions were used to report the findings.

Utilization rates are reported for the acute hospital, extended care facility and home care service. The authors pointed out that the number of discharges, days of care and average length of stay in acute hospitals was less for the over 65 population in the health plan, once the extended care and home care services were initiated. The use of such facilities, in contrast to acute hospital care, is much less costly. They concluded that this particular project had demonstrated that these services could be successfully integrated into a prepaid group practice program that already provides a range of hospital and ambulatory care services.

Hurtado, A.V., et al.

1973   "Determinants of medical care utilization: failure to keep appointments." *Med. Care* 11 (May-June): 189-198.

This study analyzes the impact of selected patient and physician characteristics on patients' failure to keep appointments in a prepaid, multispecialty group practice.

Data on a five percent sample of Kaiser Health Plan members during 1969 were collected from clinic records during that year.

Appointment failures were of two types: patients who did not appear for an appointment and did not notify the system (DNA) and people who cancelled on the same day of their appointment (cancellations).

Patient characteristics analyzed to try to explain these appointment failures were whether or not the member was a regular health plan member or a poverty group enrollee, the mean number of scheduled appointments and office visits he had, his age, sex, family size, attitudes toward Kaiser physicians, presenting symptoms, and his responses to questions about whether one should go see a doctor for selected symptoms.

Physician characteristics examined were his age and specialty.

Simple cross-tabulation of rates and percentages comprised the data analysis.

There was a high relationship between the frequency of appointments and the frequency of appointment failures. High medical utilizers were most apt to have failures. The demographic and psychosocial patient characteristics, as well as physician characteristics, were much less significant in determining patient failure to keep an appointment. The medically indigent did, however, have significantly higher rates than the regular plan membership.

Kahn, L., et al.

1973   "Patient's perceptions and uses of a pediatric emergency room." *Soc. Sci. Med.* 7 (February): 155-160.

This study was undertaken in the emergency room of the St. Louis Children's Hospital to examine the characteristics of the patients and their parents who utilize the emergency room.

A sample of patients registered in the emergency room of the hospital between May 20 and September 1, 1969, was taken. The escort (usually the mother or both parents) was interviewed. Eighteen percent (18%) of the patients were white. The rest were black. Fifty-six percent (56%) of the patients lived with both parents.

The examining physician for each patient also completed a short questionnaire indicating his opinion of the appropriateness of the visit, his estimate of the urgency of the medical condition and the medical disposition of the patient.

Information collected from the patient's escort included his race, social class, residence, regular source of care, the patient's (or his parents') perception of the severity of his illness and the factors motivating the individual to seek medical care.

Cross-tabulations of percentage distributions were used to describe the findings.

For 63 percent of those who came to the emergency room, increased concern and/or belief that the child's condition had worsened was the reason cited for coming. Belief that the illness was an emergency was cited in 18 percent of the cases. Enabling factors such as transportation or work schedules were said to account for the visit to the emergency room in only seven percent of the cases.

The escort's and physician's perceptions of the severity of the child's illness differed. The physicians considered only 68 percent of the visits to be appropriate and 32 percent inappropriate. Only ten percent of the patients were considered emergencies that required the services of the emergency room.

Kaitaranta, H. and T. Purola

     1973   "A systems-oriented approach to the consumption of medical commodities." *Soc. Sci. Med.* 7 (July): 531-540.

This study suggests a dynamic systems model to explain the factors leading to the consumption of medical commodities.

This is primarily a conceptual, rather than an empirical article. It describes the theoretical framework applied in an evaluation of universal sickness insurance in Finland.

The consumption of medical commodities is seen as part of a multiphasic process involving interactions within and between different systems — individual's psycho-biological system, the general system of nature and the general social system. The main processes that occur within and among these systems are as follows:

    1. Occurrence of a disease

2. Perception of illness
3. Perception of need for medical commodities
4. Demand for medical commodities supplied at the entrance to the health system
5. Consumption of medical commodities supplied at the entrance to the health system
6. Derived demand for medical commodities initiated by consumption at the entrance to the health system
7. Derived consumption of medical commodities initiated by derived demand.

The factors that intervene throughout these processes are of several kinds. Factor group 1 includes symptoms, beliefs, knowledge and other predisposing factors that determine whether an individual falls in a state of perceived need. Factor group 2 includes those who do not perceive, but do possess, medically defined need. Factor group 3 includes those who perceive need and initiate care. Their behavior is shaped by both predisposing and enabling (income, insurance coverage) properties. Factor group 4 contains those people who decide not to seek medical care. It describes the psychological and sociopsychological (non-medical) factors used to get rid of perceived need.

Factor 5 (F5) concerns the fit between the amount and structure of demand and the actual supply of resources. Factor 6 involves the derived demand for care, once entry is gained. Factor 7 is similar to F5, but is linked to the supply of commodities available to meet derived demand. Factor group 8 refers to the derived demand for non-medical commodities created by the derived demand for medical ones. Factor 9 means the derived consumption of non-medical commodities, such as sickness and disability insurance.

The authors emphasize the importance of considering a process-oriented approach to research on the consumption of medical and related non-medical commodities.

Keller, G.B. and M.D. Keller

1973   "Concepts of sensitivity and specificity in the evaluation of emergency medical services." *Soc. Sci. Med.* 7 (November): 861-864.

The concepts of sensitivity and specificity introduced by G. Gibson, with respect to evaluating emergency medical services are explored further.

Data are based on the authors' "general experience" with events, such as automobile accidents in median level incidence areas (500 emergency events per 100,000 persons per year).

The concept of sensitivity, in relating service to need, refers to a measure of the proportion of the individuals requiring a given service who actually receive it. Specificity, on the other hand, refers to a measure of the proportion of individuals who do not require a given service and who indeed do not receive it.

These concepts are applied to the sequence of services in emergency medical care systems.

Cross-tabulation of percentage distributions are used to report the findings.

The authors conclude that "specificity" improves at each subsequent step of rendering emergency care — call, dispatch, transport, treatment in emergency medical facility, hospitalization — as the decision makers have more first-hand information to go by.

Lefcowitz, M.J.

> 1973   "Poverty and health: a re-examination." *Inquiry* 10
>   (March): 3-13.

This article re-examines the relationship between poverty and health and the utilization of medical services.

Data from the National Center for Health Statistics on morbidity, mortality and the utilization of health services are reviewed.

The utilization indices examined were number of physician visits per person per year, percent using selected types of specialists and site of the visit.

Use was examined by occupation, income level, race, years of schooling, degree of chronic activity limitation and prevalence of selected disease conditions.

The author argues that when education is taken into account in analyzing the relationship between income and the utilization indices, the correlation is considerably diminished. Further, taking age into account, he contends there is very little relationship between income and the prevalence of chronic conditions. He offers explanations of the impact of education on use in terms of differing life styles of the better and least educated and the effects of permanent income, for which education is a proxy. He does concede that in economic terms, however, the costs of illness are inequitably distributed among the income categories and, hence, may cause or increase impoverishment.

Levenson, I.

1972   "Access to medical care: the Queensbridge Experiment." *Inquiry* 9 (June): 61-68.

The purpose of this study is to analyze the factors that influenced whether or not persons registered for a health maintenance organization.

Data were collected from a sample of 1,219 of approximately 1,400 residents age 60 and over of the Queensbridge Housing Project, Long Island, New York, between January 1963 and fall, 1964.

The number who registered for services through the Queensbridge Health Maintenance Service (QHMS) served as the utilization index.

The variables analyzed were age, sex, color, self-rating of health, mobility level, travel time, health insurance, usual source of care, income, marital status, number in household, education, employment status, length of residence, foreign-born and religion.

Dummy variable regression, the F-test and Chi-square test of statistical significance were used to analyze the data.

Health status was a major determinant of whether people registered. Income was a powerful determinant, also. The more educated and recent residents of the area appear more likely to use the clinic services. When other variables were held constant, color was not important. Jewish residents were more likely to use the clinic, however. A "discouraging finding" the author cited was the low utilization rate by persons lacking an alternative source of care. These data suggest, concludes the author, that patients will not be attracted by an efficient entry point to what they perceive to be the same unsatisfactory services.

Li, F.P., et al.

1972   "Health care for the Chinese community in Boston." *Amer. J. Public Health* 62 (April): 536-539.

This report discusses some of the social and cultural reasons for the underutilization of community health facilities by Chinese-Americans, particularly those who have recently emigrated to the United States.

Analysis of secondary data on the utilization of health services by Chinese-Americans provided the information for this report.

The report discusses the "underutilization" of health services by Chinese-Americans, but does not provide a precise empirical definition of "underutilization."

The relationship of cultural beliefs, lack of information about available health facilities and insurance programs and the inability to speak English well to health level and use by Chinese-Americans was described.

The authors concluded that many Chinese-American communities have poor health standards and a high incidence of disease. They tend to underutilize because of their cultural beliefs about health and illness and their distrust of Western medical practices and physicians. They also underutilize because of their poverty and their lack of knowledge about health insurance plans and free clinics.

Loewenstein, R.

1971　　"Early effects of Medicare on the health care of the aged." *Soc. Sec. Bull.* 34 (April): 3-20; 42.

This article reports patterns in use of hospital and medical care by persons aged 65 and over and in charges for such services both before and after the implementation of Medicare.

In April and May of 1966 a nationwide sample of social security beneficiaries aged 65 and over were interviewed about their use of health services in the previous year. In November and December, 1967, persons in a comparable but independent sample were interviewed about their experiences during the previous year under Medicare.

Information was reported on the hospitalization rates, charges, and length of stay by type of facility; the percent with visits, mean number of visits and place of visit for ambulatory medical encounters; and total charges and charges per person for medical services overall.

The utilization and cost information was reported by age, sex, race, region, residence, family size, family income, type of insurance coverage, and whether or not surgery was performed.

Cross-tabulation of rates were used to report the findings.

For short-stay hospital care, the most significant change occurred in the days of care per aged person, which rose 25 percent. Significantly larger increases were noted for certain segments of the aged population — including persons 75 and over, nonwhites, residents in the South, persons in urban areas outside SMSA's and persons in one-member family units with low incomes.

Before Medicare, a substantial portion of hospital stays — 17 percent — was without charges incurred; under Medicare the percent was reduced to three percent. The rate of hospital days with charges rose 50 percent but was doubled for persons 75 and over and nonwhites.

The proportion of total hospital charges paid out-of-pocket declined from 38 percent to seven percent (7%).

There was a shift from the use of nursing homes to extended care facilities that provide a higher level of skilled nursing. Out-of-pocket expenditures for care in these long-term institutions decreased from 98 percent of charges before Medicare to 80 percent after Medicare.

Medicare seemed to result in a shift from clinic and home visits to office visits. No significant changes, however, were found in the proportion who had ambulatory visits, and a slight decrease was noted in the mean number of visits per person.

Total out-of-pocket expenses for medical services decreased from 81 percent to 47 percent of the total charges. Medicare apparently had no effect on the average charges for services. There were substantial increases in total institutional charges for care, however.

Mechanic, D.

1972   *Public Expectations and Health Care: Essays on the Changing Organization of Health Services.* New York: John Wiley and Sons.

This book of essays is an overview of many of the issues involved with the organization, utilization and satisfaction with the health care system.

Selected data from secondary sources in the United States and England are cited.

The context of health care is examined in terms of the expected goals of the system and how it has been affected by developments in the growth of government involvement, social forces affecting the maintenance of health and the prevention of disease, and the organization of the medical profession.

The character and distribution of health services is described in the context of the various social functions of medical care, health services utilization and how medicine can be more responsive to the needs of patients. Special emphasis is placed on the problems of the low-income and the potential of prepaid group practice plans for improving access to care.

The National Health Service in Britain is analyzed to stimulate insights into some of the dilemmas that face the American health care system. Special issues in health care the author considers include the manner in which patients come to define illness, the use of medical facilities, response to treatment, the relationships between social psychological factors and the onset of illness, etc.

The author concludes with a summary of the current state of affairs in the United States and suggestions for improving the distribution and training of physicians and ultimately the quality of care rendered.

Miller, M.H.

1973   "Seeking advice for cancer symptoms." *Amer. J. Public Health* 63 (November): 955-961.

This study examined individuals' utilization of lay referral systems prior to consulting a physician for a particular symptom.

A sample of 139 patients from a Head and Neck Cancer Clinic were interviewed.

Individuals were asked to list all the people they had consulted for their symptom before seeing a doctor, and whether they had accepted or rejected the advice given by this "lay referral system."

Respondents were grouped into three social classes — lower, middle and upper.

Cross-tabulation of percentage distributions was used to analyze the data.

The author concluded that the "professional practitioner is but one consultant of many, and the patient often arrives at his office after having exhausted a whole network of less formal consultants." The author drew several generalizations from the findings:

1) Respondents in the upper and middle classes were more likely to consult only with their spouses, while lower class respondents often consulted friends and neighbors, also, before seeing a doctor.

2) Respondents who did not seek advice from others and hence, lacked the support and reassurance of others, delayed longer in obtaining professional care than those who did consult a lay referral network.

3) Lower-class respondents followed lay advice more often than those in the upper and middle classes.

4) Contrary to E. Freidson's contentions, a "lay referral structure" involves medically informed (i.e., a nurse, or pharmacist) as well as medically-uninformed individuals.

Miller, M.H.

1973   "Who receives optimal care?" *J. Health Soc. Behav.* 14 (June): 176-182.

This study re-evaluates the assumption that upper class individuals receive more effective care than those of the lower class.

A sample of patients with head and neck cancer who were referred to a State-funded cancer research center by their physician from January, 1969 to February, 1970, were interviewed.

Respondents were asked how long they used a physician before being referred to the specialist at the center, and why they changed from one practitioner to another — by their own choice or on the suggestion of their physician.

The social class of the respondents — lower, middle or upper — was determined from Hollingshead's Index of Social Position.

Cross-tabulation of percent distributions were used to analyze the data.

The authors concluded that upper-class individuals received more personalized care from their physicians, in that the physician attempted to treat the patient for a long period of time before referring him to a specialist. The upper-class individuals, thus, had a closer interpersonal relationship with their physician and greater continuity of care.

On the other hand, lower- and middle-class individuals received less personalized treatment but more rapid referral to the specialists at the clinic and thus, faster access to the special care necessary to their disease.

Montiero, L.A.

1973   "Expense is no object . . . income and physician visits reconsidered." *J. Health Soc. Behav.* 14 (June): 99-115.

This article re-examines the relationship between income and physician visits, especially the assumption that the poor underutilize physician services.

Interviews with samples of 1,100 residents of Rhode Island over a three year period (1967, 1968, 1969) yielded the data. Information from the National Center for Health Statistics was also presented.

The total number of physician visits per year was the use index reported.

Characteristics for which use was analyzed included the age, race, income level, pro-physician orientation, source of health care and source of insurance coverage of respondents.

Cross-tabulation of percentage distributions were used to report the findings.

This article argues that there is no longer a clear-cut difference between income groups with respect to their use of physician services. There is a "bimodal distribution" of physician use by income now, i.e., those whose income is under $3,000 or over $10,000 have equal rates of physician visits. The factors which seemed to give rise to these utilization patterns were 1) the need for services because of illness, and 2) the availability of publicly financed medical care. There is an equal tendency, say the authors, for various income groups to visit physicians when ill. But since lower income groups report more illness (in part, because many in these groups are aged) this increased need is reflected in higher use rates. Lower income respondents who have publicly-financed care through Medicaid, etc. also use more physician services than the high-income, who do not have the benefit of such coverage.

Moore, G.T., et al.

> 1972   "Effect of a neighborhood health center on hospital
>   emergency room use." *Med. Care* 2 (May-June):
>   240-247.

The purpose of this study is to examine the impact of a neighborhood health center on the use of the hospital emergency room.

A random sample of ten percent of the individuals who were users of either the emergency room or the new neighborhood health center associated with Massachusetts General Hospital were selected to be interviewed. The year before the center opened was the control year and the first two years of the operation of the center the study years.

The study attempted to assess if there was a decrease in the use of emergency room (ER) facilities for other than true emergencies.

Cross-tabulation of percentage distributions of ER utilization before and after the introduction of the center were reported.

The study showed that there was no decrease in emergency room utilization after the opening of the neighborhood health center. However, those individuals who were registered with the center seemed to use the emergency room only for emergencies, or when the center was closed. They did, therefore, use the emergency room less for non-urgent presenting complaints than did those who were not registered. The authors conclude that after a few years, more people may register at and use the center, and subsequent decrease in utilization of the ER will occur.

Moroney, R.M. and N. Kurtz

> 1973 "Extended care benefits: a comparison of utilization of two age groups." *Inquiry* 10 (March): 50-53.

This study examines the potential of the extended care facility (ECF) as a viable alternative to the hospital for the total population — not just for the aged.

The data were a part of a larger study comparing the utilization experiences of two populations, who were covered either by Medicare or the United Auto Workers (UAW). The UAW plan is similar to Medicare in intent, but has a larger benefit package. Data came from three sources: patient interviews, nursing home records, and records from the fiscal intermediaries. The study was conducted in Detroit, during 1968-1970.

The percent of ECF patients receiving services in the over 65 and under 65 age groups were compared, as were the mean number of services they received.

The two age groups were quite similar in terms of selected social characteristics — sex, religion, education and family size. The older groups were somewhat less apt to be married, however. Those 65 and over reported more while those under 65 reported diseases of the central nervous system.

Cross-tabulations were used to report the data.

The authors concluded that when an extended care benefit package was provided to all age groups, those who actually used the benefits tended to be aged. Very few people under 45 years of age used the benefit, while 87 percent of all users were 50 years or older. Such a finding is probably accounted for the greater number of diagnoses reported by the elderly.

Mott, F.D., et al.

> 1973 "Prepaid group practice in Sault Ste. Marie, Ontario: Part II. evidence from the household survey." *Med. Care* 11 (May-June): 173-188.

This article reports a second phase of the study of the different utilization patterns of Canadian steelworkers enrolled in a prepaid group practice plan and those who got care from independent practitioners through an indemnity plan.

Household interviews were used to collect data from samples of Canadian steelworker union enrollees in the Group Health Association

(GHA) and the Indemnification Insurance Plan (IIP). The study was conducted July 1, 1967 through June 30, 1968. The data obtained through interviews reported here and the clinical record information described in an earlier study seemed to agree quite closely.

The utilization information analyzed included the number and percent distribution of physician visits related to acute illness, injury, or chronic conditions during the two-week period preceding the interview, site of visit, type of practitioner seen, usual doctor, pattern of referral, hospital discharges, length of stay, and days of care per 1000 persons per year.

These measures were reported and compared for the GHA and IIP samples. The rates were analyzed by the sex of the respondents, the experience of restricted activity or bed disability days, acute illness or injury, or chronic conditions, "symptom/condition" complexes, surgery, diagnoses, and immunization levels.

The data were reported in terms of cross-tabulation of percent distributions and rates.

The two study populations were quite similar demographically. There were no clean-cut statistical differences between them in the incidence of acute illness, prevalence of chronic disease, disability due to acute or chronic illness, the prevalence of symptom/condition complexes, or immunization levels among children. Identical or very similar findings were reported for medical attendance in acute illness, medical services for symptom/conditions, and reasons for not seeking care for the latter.

The Group Health Centre of GHA was clearly the "medical care home base" for those enrollees, as evidenced by concentration of services there and lower use of hospital outpatient and other facilities. The continuity of care, expressed in patterns of referrals and having a usual doctor was higher for IIP members. Hospital discharges were about 25 percent higher for the IIP group than for GHA, with utilization of days of hospital care also higher and surgery being responsible for a substantial part of the difference.

Murnaghan, J.H.

1973   "Review of the Conference (on Ambulatory Medical Care Records) Proceedings." *Med. Care* 11 (March-April Supplement): 13-34.

This conference addressed many of the issues that are relevant to consider in evaluating "access."

The conference emphasized the importance of knowing the population-at-risk for a given delivery system. Household surveys of these populations provide information about the users and non-users of health services in an area.

Conference participants identified three dimensions that are important for appraising the access of the population to the system: 1) measures of entry into a system of care, reflecting accessibility and availability of services; 2) measures of quality of care once the patient is in the system, including structure, process and outcome, and 3) measures of exit from the system, involving satisfaction, compliance, and general acceptability of the services provided.

McDonald, A.D., et al.

1973   "Physician service in Montreal before universal health insurance." *Med. Care* 11 (July-August): 269-286.

This article reports the results of three surveys conducted during 1969-70 as part of the first phase of a before and after study of the introduction of comprehensive health insurance in the Montreal metropolitan area.

A survey of a random sample of 6,000 households over a 12-month period, interviews with a random sample of 497 practicing doctors in Montreal, between October 1969 and May 1970, and interviews with 1,766 patients who attended emergency rooms in six Montreal hospitals for reasons other than an accident within 24 hours and with 1,694 who attended outpatient departments in two hospitals, provided the data.

Mean physician visits and the proportion with symptoms and the proportion who saw a doctor were analyzed by age, family size and family income from the household survey data.

The distribution of physicians' working time by site, the time spent with patients and the percent employing ancillary personnel and the mean hours they worked were reported from the survey of physicians.

Information on the urgency of presenting complaints, usual source of care, and source of referral were collected in the surveys of emergency room and outpatient department users.

Cross-tabulation of percentage distributions and rates were used to analyze the data.

The results of the household survey showed that after family income was adjusted for family size, a direct relationship existed between income and use of physician services. The relationship was particularly strong for children. It was also found that low-income people had more unmet need, judging by the proportion with symptoms and the proportion who contacted a physician in each income group.

The average working day for physicians ranged from 9.7 hours for general internists to 11.7 hours for psychiatrists. The number of patients seen, excluding telephone consultations, ranged from 70 patients per week for psychiatrists to 140 patients per week for general practitioners. Ancillary help of some kind was employed by 73 percent of general practitioners and 90 percent of the specialists.

The majority (83 percent) of the emergency room patients interviewed had non-urgent conditions. Of those attending the two outpatient departments, 61 percent claimed this as their usual source of care, and 70 percent came without referral from a physician. While 70 percent thought that continuity of care was important, two-thirds said they would prefer the outpatient department even if all medical care was free.

The three surveys were repeated in 1971-72, approximately one year after the introduction of comprehensive health insurance in Montreal.

McKinlay, J.B.

    1973   "Social networks, lay consultation and help-seeking
               behavior." *Social Forces* 51 (March): 275-292.

This article examines the role of the family, its kin and friendship networks in the use of health and welfare services.

Eighty-seven working-class families (consisting of two subsamples of "utilizing" and "underutilizing" respondents) were studied in Aberdeen, Scotland, over a period of roughly one and a half years.

A woman was regarded as a "utilizer" if she: (a) attended the Aberdeen City Maternity Clinic for her first antenatal visit before the end of the seventeenth week of gestation, and (b) having had her pregnancy confirmed by the obstetric staff, attended regularly for antenatal care. A woman was an "underutilizer if she: (a) had no antenatal preparation, or (b) attended for some form of care only after the twenty-eighth week of gestation, or (c) was an emergency admission during labor without any previous prenatal care, or (d) defaulted from her clinic appointments more than three times consecutively without offering an excuse.

Information was collected on the sample's kin and friendship networks, socio-economic status, parity, education level, proximity to services and length of residence in the city.

A Chi-square test of significance was used to analyze the data.

After controlling for the socio-economic and other related variables, differences were found between the utilizers and underutilizers on various aspects of their social networks. The underutilizers relied on an undifferentiated group of readily available relatives and friends as lay consultants before using the service. Utilizers, however, appeared to both differentiate between relatives and friends, and be independent of both these sources of social control. The author then summarizes the implications of these findings for help-seeking behavior.

McKinlay, J.B. and S.M. McKinlay

1972   "Some social characteristics of lower working class utilizers and underutilizers of maternity care services." *J. Health Soc. Behav.* 13 (December): 369-392.

This study was intended to explain the factors that affect the utilization of maternity services by lower working class mothers.

Eighty-seven unskilled working class families — consisting of two sub-samples of "utilizing" and "under-utilizing" respondents drawn from a hospital-based maternity clinic in Aberdeen, Scotland — were interviewed four times over a period of roughly one and a half years to collect the data.

A woman was regarded as a utilizer if she (a) attended the clinic for her first antenatal visit before the end of the seventeenth week of gestation, and (b) attended regularly for subsequent antenatal care. Underutilizers were those who (a) had no antenatal preparation, or (b) attended only after the twenty-eighth week of gestation, or (c) was an emergency admission during labor without any previous prenatal care, or (d) if she failed to appear for appointments more than three times without notifying the clinic.

The variables that were used to describe respondents were as follows: present age, age at first conception, legal status of first pregnancy, total number of pregnancies recorded, marital status, attitude toward present pregnancy, present marital status of parents, household composition, status of household ownership, parents' residential mobility, number of schools attended, moving rate, husband's employment stability, overtime and type of employment, and the respondent's and respondent's mother's employment status.

Percent distributions were used to describe the findings.

The authors conclude that underutilizers, more so than utilizers, appear to sustain a crisis existence. They experience lack of permanent accommodation, over-crowding marital instability, financial difficulties, and frequent sickness in the family. Utilizers appear to avoid most of these problems. Further, the circumstances surrounding the first conception (whether or not it is legitimate) appear to distinguish who is apt to be a utilizer and who a crisis-oriented underutilizer.

NCHS

1971   *Persons Hospitalized by Number of Hospital Episodes and Days in Year:* Series 10. Number 64.

Statistics on persons with one or more episodes in short-stay hospitals during an average year, according to number of episodes, days hospitalized, and patterns of stay, based on 1968 Health Interview Survey, are reported.

There were 18.7 million people hospitalized in 1968. This represents a rate of 96 persons hospitalized per 1,000 population. Hospitalization for males increased with advancing age. This pattern was not true for females, due to the higher hospitalization rates for women in the child-bearing ages 15-44.

About 85.7 percent of the people had only one hospital episode during th year; 14.4 percent had multiple episodes. Those with multiple episodes were more apt to be those with low family incomes, living outside SMSA's, aged 65 and over, females, or white persons.

The most common pattern of hospital stay was a single episode of one to seven days. The average length of stay per person hospitalized was 10.4 days. Females age 15-44 had lower average lengths of stay because of hospitalizations for childbirth.

NCHS

1972   *Age Patterns in Medical Care, Illness, and Disability: United States – 1968-1969.* Series 10. Number 70.

Statistics on the use of medical services and the extent of illness and disability in the population by age, with emphasis on the health status of persons 65 years and over, based on the Health Interview Survey during 1968-1969, are reported.

White persons had a higher rate of hospital discharges but a shorter length of stay than did all other persons. Lower income groups had a higher rate of hospitalization and longer lengths of stay. Males had lower rate of physician visits than females at all ages except for persons under 17. About 69 percent of the population had had a physician visit during the year prior to the interview and only 45 percent had had a dental visit.

About two out of five persons 65 years and over reported chronic activity limitation. In general, as persons advanced in age the number of injuries they incurred decreased. Approximately 60 percent of all injuries among persons 65 years and over occurred in the home.

NCHS

1972   *Current Estimates from the Health Interview Survey: United States — 1970.* Series 10. Number 72.

This report presents provisional estimates of the incidence of acute conditions, number of persons reporting activity limitation, number of persons injured, hospital discharges, persons with hospital episodes, disability days, and frequency of dental and physician visits, based on data collected from the 1970 Health Interview Survey.

The findings on health services utilization will be summarized in some detail. The number of discharges from short-stay hospitals was 13.3 per 100 persons in 1970. The average length of stay was 8.6 days — 10.0 for males and 7.6 for females. About 10.3 percent of the population had one hospital episode. The majority had only *one* episode.

There was an average of 1.5 dentist visits per person in 1970. The percent who had at least one dentist visit was 46.8 percent. About 12.7 percent of the population had never seen a dentist.

There were an average of 4.6 physician visits per person in 1970. Approximately 71.9 percent of the population had at least one physician contact in 1970.

NCHS

1972   *Home Care for Persons 55 Years and Over: United States –July 1966-June 1968.* Series 10. Number 73.

Statistics on persons 55 years and over receiving care at home by selected demographic characteristics, type of care received, type of condition, duration of care, and providers of care, based on data collected in the Health Interview Survey from July 1966 through June 1968 are reported.

Persons receiving home care represented a 4.9 percent of the population 55 or over during the interview period. About 86.1 percent of the persons receiving home care received personal care — help in moving about, dressing, bath and eating. Approximately 26.6 percent received medically related care — changing bandages, injections, etc.

The proportion of the population reporting home care increased with age. Proportionately more females received care than males. More persons with annual incomes of less than $5,000 received home care than did persons with higher incomes. Relatively fewer white persons than nonwhites received home care.

The main condition for which personal care was provided was for arthritis and rheumatism. Diabetes was the main condition for which medical treatment was rendered.

The majority of care was provided by family members residing in the household (79.8 percent). Registered nurses provided care to 7.0 percent.

The introduction of Medicare during the survey period probably accounted for a decline in the percent receiving care at home from 1966-67 to 1967-68.

NCHS

1972   *Health Characteristics of Low-Income Persons.* Series 10. Number 74.

This report is an analysis of the health characteristics of persons with family incomes under $5,000 and a comparison of aid recipients with nonrecipients. Based on data from the 1968 Health Interview Survey, the report describes the population in terms of status, demographic characteristics, comparative health status, type and extent of disability, medical care and hospitalization.

Persons with incomes of less than $5,000 have more activity limitation, more disability, and more hospital episodes than the total population. Unfortunately, they have fewer resources for obtaining medical care: fewer have hospital insurance and, by definition, they have less cash to pay for medical expenses. Within the low-income group, aid recipients have poorer health than nonrecipients. Of all health measures, they have higher rates than nonrecipients — in many cases, twice as high. Persons receiving aid averaged more visits to a physician and were more likely to see him in his office than nonrecipients. The majority or visits by both recipients and nonrecipients were made to general practitioners for diagnosis or treatment of illness, rather than preventive care.

NCHS

1972   *Physician Visits — Volume and Interval Since Last Visit: United States–1969.* Series 10. Number 75.

This report presents statistics on the time interval since last physician visit, the volume of physician visits, and the number of visits per person per year by selected demographic characteristics. Also presented are statistics on the number of physician visits by place of visit, type of service, condition causing visit for diagnosis and treatment, length of time to get to the physician, and waiting time at place of visit, based on the 1969 Health Interview Survey.

An estimated 69.4 percent of the population reported having seen or talked to a physician for medical advice at least once in the survey year. There were an average of 4.3 visits per person during the year. The average number of visits were higher for females than males, for those 65 or older, whites, those with 13 or more years of schooling, residents of SMSA's, people who live in the West, and those who were unable to carry on their major activity. In contrast to previous years, in 1969 the low-income averaged slightly more physician visits (4.8) than the high-income (4.5).

About 70.1 percent of the physician visits during 1969 took place in the doctor's office, 12.0 percent were by telephone, and 10.3 percent were in a hospital clinic or emergency room. About 59.2 percent of all visits were to general practitioners. The second largest group of visits was to pediatricians (9.3 percent). About 75 percent of all visits were for diagnosis and treatment of a condition. An estimated 44.9 percent of the conditions were chronic and 48.8 percent acute. The average length of time for patients to get to the doctor's office was 17.2 minutes. If the patient had an appointment, he waited an estimated 30.4 minutes in the doctor's office before he was seen.

NCHS

1972   *Dental Visits — Volume and Interval Since Last Visit: United States-1969.* Series 10. Number 76.

This report presents statistics on the volume of dental visits and the time interval since the last dental visit by age, sex, color, family income, education of the head of the family, usual activity status, place of residence and geographic region, based on the 1969 Health Interview Survey.

During 1969 about 45.0 percent of the population had at least one visit to a dentist. There were an average of 1.5 visits per person during the year.

The number of dentist visits per person per year was highest in the age group 5-24. The rate was higher for females than males, for whites than nonwhites and for high-income than for low-income. The average number of visits was greater for those persons in families where the head was well-educated, for metropolitan residents, and for residents of the Northeast and West than for residents of the North Central and South Regions.

NCHS

1972   *Use of Special Aids: United States-1969.* Series 10. Number 78.

Statistics on the distribution and use of artificial limbs, braces, crutches, canes, special shoes, wheelchairs, walkers and other special aids for getting around, based on data collected from the 1969 Health Interview Survey, are reported.

An estimated 3.2 percent of the population used one or more types of special aids. Persons 15-44 reported the lowest percentage use of aids (1.2 percent) and persons 65 or older the highest percent (13.3 percent). Males had higher proportionate use of one or more aids than did females at all ages under 65. The reverse was true for those 65 or older.

A slightly higher percentage of whites and persons with family incomes under $5,000 used special aids. Persons living alone or with nonrelatives had greater proportionate use of special aids than did family members. Usually working persons had the lowest percentage with special aids. Increased severity of activity limitation was associated with the use of aids.

NCHS

1973   *Current Estimates from the Health Interview Survey: United States-1971.* Series 10. Number 79.

This report provides provisional estimates of the incidence of acute conditions, number of persons reporting activity limitation, number of persons injured, hospital discharges, persons with hospital episodes, disability days, and frequency of dental and physician visits, based on the 1971 Health Interview Survey.

The findings on utilization will be summarized in some detail. There were an estimated 13.6 discharges per 100 persons in 1971. The average length of stay in 1971 was 8.5 days. Approximately 10.5 percent had one or more hospital episodes. About 84 percent had only one hospitalization.

The average number of dentist visits was 1.5. Approximately 47 percent of the population had at least one dentist visit. Approximately 30 percent of all dental visits were for fillings, 12.3 percent for extractions and fillings, 18 percent for cleaning and 13 percent for dentures.

There were 4.9 visits to a physician per person in 1971. Approximately 72 percent saw a medical doctor at least once in 1971.

NCHS

1973   *Volume of X-Ray Visits: United States — April-September 1970.* Series 10. Number 81.

This report provides statistics on the volume of medical and dental x-ray visits, by area of body x-rayed, place of x-ray visit, type of x-ray, age, sex, race, place of residence, geographic region, family income and education, based on data collected in the 1970 Health Interview Survey.

The average number of medical x-ray visits per 100 persons increased with age, while persons 15-24 years of age had the highest rate of dental x-rays. Males and females had medical x-rays at similar rates, but females were more likely to have dental x-rays than males. Whites had more medical *and* dental x-rays than nonwhites. The rate of dental x-rays rose with family income, whereas the population with less family income had more medical x-ray visits.

Increases in population density and educational attainment of the family head produced higher rates of medical and dental x-ray visits. The population in the West reported more x-rays for both medical and dental purposes than did people in the Northeast, North Central, and South Regions.

The major area of the body x-rayed was the chest. The hospital was the major place in which x-rays were made.

NCHS

1972   *Nursing Homes: Their Admission Policies, Admissions, and Discharges: United States — April-September 1968.* Series 12. Number 16.

Statistics on the number and types of nursing and related care homes according to admission policies, total admissions, admissions according to the former place of residence, total discharges, discharges alive and due to death, rate of patient turnover, and length of stay were reported, based on the 1968 Nursing Home Survey.

The percent of the total number of homes accepting patients with physical problems range from 67.0 percent for postsurgical recovery patients to 88.2 percent for persons with heart disease. Fifty-two and six-tenths percent (52.6 percent) of the homes accepted mentally retarded patients and 23.7 percent accepted alcoholics. Most nursing and related care homes (83.2 percent) required that all persons admitted to the home be examined by a physician.

The most common former places of residence for persons admitted were general hospitals and patients' homes. Of the 756,289 discharges from nursing and related care homes, 29.5 percent were because of death. The highest rate of patient turnover during the survey year occurred in nursing homes, probably due to the enactment of Medicare, which emphasizes the discharge of patients within 100 days. The length of stay was shorter in nursing homes, for homes that were proprietary and in larger homes.

NCHS

1972   *Services and Activities Offered to Nursing Home Residents: United States-1968.* Series 12. Number 17.

Statistics on rehabilitation services, recreational activities, and arrangements for physician services provided to nursing home residents, by type of nursing service and bed size of home and number of employees are presented from data collected in the 1968 Nursing Home Survey.

Of the 19,533 nursing homes in 1968, only seven percent had a full-time staff physician, and only 34 percent arranged for a physician to visit at regular intervals. Only 32 percent offered rehabilitative services. Half of the 813,335 residents in nursing homes were in homes not providing rehabilitative services. Some of the homes that did not offer rehabilitation programs sent their residents to outpatient care clinics instead.

Although 15,443 nursing homes (79 percent) offered recreational activities, the more extensive activities — arts/crafts and trips — were offered in only 7,585 and 4,989 homes respectively. In homes that offered recreational activities, only 21 percent employed a recreational therapist.

NCHS

1973   *Characteristics of Residents in Nursing and Per-*

sonal Care Homes: United States-June-August 1969. Series 12. Number 19.

This report presents statistics on residents in nursing and personal care homes during July-August 1969 by age, color, sex, region, type of care, type of ownership, length of stay, and marital status, based on the 1969 Resident Places Survey.

About 89 percent of the residents of nursing and personal care homes were age 65 and over, 32 percent were age 85 and over. More than two-thirds (69.1 percent) were females and the vast majority (95.5 percent) white. The largest proportion of the residents (35 percent) were in the North Central Region. The majority of the residents (78 percent) were in homes where the primary service was nursing care. Government-owned homes had a much larger proportion of patients under 65. The average length of stay for all residents was just under three years; the average was slightly higher for females. Sixty-two percent (62 percent) of the residents were widowed. Residents who were married at the time of admission had spent less time in the homes than those who were in the other marital status categories.

NCHS

1973   *Charges for Care and Sources of Payment for Residents in Nursing Homes: United States-June-August 1969.* Series 12. Number 21.

Data on charges for care and sources of payment for nursing home residents in relation to service, ownership, geographic region of the nursing home and age, sex, and health status of the resident are presented, based on the 1969 Resident Places Survey.

Residents in homes providing nursing care paid significantly more per month ($356) than residents paid in homes providing personal care ($178). Charges for those 65 or over were greater than for those under 65. Rates for males and females were quite similar. Residents receiving intensive nursing care paid higher charges than did residents receiving no nursing or personal care. Charges varied by diagnoses and the number of chronic conditions reported by the patient. Over three-fourths of the residents used their own or family income or public assistance other than Medicare or Medicaid as the primary source of payment.

NCHS

1971   *Utilization of Short-Stay Hospitals — Summary of
            Non-Medical Statistics: United States-1966.* Series
            13. Number 8.

This report presents statistics on the utilization of short-stay hospitals based on data collected in the Hospital Discharge Survey from a national sample of hospital records of discharged patients in 1966.

Discharges, days of care, and average length of stay are distributed by each of the following variables — age, sex, color, geographical region, hospital bed size, and type of hospital ownership.

An estimated 28.8 million inpatients were discharged from short-stay hospitals during 1966. There were 150 discharges and 1,221 inpatient days per 1,000. Average length of stay was 8.1 days.

The discharge rate for all patients under one year of age (232.5 per 1,000) was higher than the rate for any other age group under 65. This was due to discharges of nonwell newborn infants. The number of hospital discharges for persons 65 and over was 6.7 percent higher in 1966 than 1965. The average length of hospital stay increased with advancing age.

The discharge rate for females (125.3 per 1,000) was approximately 43 percent higher than that for males (123.0 per 1,000). The inclusion of admissions for deliveries lowered the average length of stay of females 15-44 years of age. When deliveries were excluded, males and females averaged similar lengths of stay.

The data on discharge rates and length of stay by color are difficult to interpret because of the large number of patients for which color was not reported.

The number of discharges in 1966 ranged from 4.6 million in the West to 9.1 million in the South. The average length of stay was generally higher in the Northeast and North Central Regions.

The largest differences in discharge rates and average length of stay by hospital size were for people 65 years of age or older. The proportion of aged patients discharged ranged from 15.2 percent in hospitals with 500 beds or more to 19.8 percent in hospitals with fewer than 100 beds. The proportion of total hospital days provided the elderly ranged from 23.9 percent in hospitals with 500 beds or more to 34.7 percent in hospitals with less than 100 beds.

Voluntary nonprofit hospitals accounted for 72 percent of all discharges, government hospitals for 20 percent and length of stay was consistently shorter in proprietary hospitals.

NCHS

1972   *Utilization of Short-Stay Hospitals — Summary of
Nonmedical Statistics: United States-1967.* Series
13. Number 9.

This report presents statistics on the utilization of short-stay hospitals based on data abstracted by the Hospital Discharge Survey in 1967.

Discharges, days of care, and average length of stay are reported by age, sex, and color of the discharged patients and by geographic region, bed size, and type of ownership of hospitals.

An estimated 28.4 million inpatients were discharged from non-Federal short-stay hospitals during 1967. These were 146.9 discharges and 1,238.9 days care per 1,000 population. The average length of stay was 8.4 days.

The discharge rates ranged from 74.8 per 1,000 population under 15 to 289.1 per 1,000 population aged 65 and over. Average length of stay increased with each successive age group.

Rates of discharge were higher for females than males. When admissions for delivery were excluded, the discharge rate for females was only 13 percent higher than for males and the average length of stay the same.

Though the findings must be interpreted with caution, because of the large number in the sample for which color was not reported, white discharge rates outnumbered nonwhites' 8 to 1. Although the average length of stay was about the same overall, in each age group and by sex, the average stay was shorter for whites than nonwhites.

Discharges by region ranged from 131.8 per 1,000 in the Northwest to 160.2 in the North Central Region. The average length of stay was shortest in the West (7.0 days) and longest in the Northeast (9.8 days).

Average length of stay increased as hospital size increased — ranging from 7.5 days in hospitals with 6-99 beds to 10.3 days in hospitals with 500 beds or more.

Voluntary nonprofit hospitals cared for the most patients and provided the largest number of days of care. The average length of stay was shortest in proprietary hospitals.

Increased hospital utilization by the aged following the institution of Medicare was the outstanding change that occurred during 1965-1967.

NCHS

1972   *Inpatient Utilization of Short-Stay Hospitals in
Each Geographic Region: United States-1966-68.*
Series 13. Number 10.

Statistics are presented on the utilization of short-stay hospitals by region based on data collected in the Hospital Discharge Survey.

Discharges, discharge rates, days of care, and average length of stay are distributed by age and sex according to geographic divisions for the calendar years 1966-1968.

The largest increase in the number of discharges was in the South Atlantic Division and the largest decrease in the West South Central. New England was the only division to have a decrease in the number of discharges 65 years of age or older. All of the divisions had a decrease in the discharge rate from 1966 to 1968 for females, including deliveries.

The largest increase in the number of days of care was in the South Atlantic, which also had the largest increase in the number of days of care for discharges 65 or over. The East South Central and the Pacific Divisions were the only ones in which there was a decrease in the average length of stay for either sex group.

NCHS

1973   *Inpatient Utilization of Short-Stay Hospitals by Diagnosis: United States-1968.* Series 13. Number 12.

Statistics are presented on the utilization of short-stay non-federal hospitals based on data abstracted by the Hospital Discharge Survey in 1968.

The number of discharges, discharge rates, and average length of stay are shown for categories of first-listed diagnoses, by demographic characteristics of inpatients and geographic region of hospitals.

Deliveries and complications of childbirth and the puerperium were the leading causes of hospitalization in 1968. Of the nonobstetrical conditions, hypertrophy of tonsils and adenoids and arteriosclerotic heart disease were the most frequently reported diagnoses. Obstetrical conditions also accounted for the most days of care. Measured by days of care, other important diagnostic groups were malignant neoplasms, fractures, vascular lesions of central nervous system, and pneumonia.

A leading cause of hospitalization by sex was arteriosclerotic heart disease for men and obstetrical conditions for women.

The most frequently reported disease for those under 15 years of age were respiratory system diseases, obstetrical conditions for those aged 15-44, digestive system diseases for those aged 45-64, and circulatory diseases for those aged 65 and over.

For whites, diseases of the digestive system ranked first and deliveries and complications of pregnancies second among the diagnostic classes in number of patients discharged. For nonwhites, obstetrical conditions and injuries were the first and second-ranking diagnostic classes.

Deliveries and complications of pregnancy ranked first in all geographic regions except the South, where a large number of persons were hospitalized for diseases of the digestive system.

NCHS

1973   *Average Length of Stay in Short-Stay Hospitals — Demographic Factors: United States-1968.* Series 13. Number 13.

Statistics are presented on the utilization of short-stay hospitals based on data collected in the 1968 Hospital Discharge Survey.

Average length of stay is presented by patient characteristics of age, sex, marital status, and color and for patients with deliveries in conjunction with hospital characteristics of size, ownership or control, and geographic region in which it is located.

The older the patient, the longer the average length of stay. Deliveries shortened the average length of stay of those 15-44 years of age. Unmarried patients over 14 years of age had longer lengths of stay than the married. Though generalizations must be made with caution, it appears that white persons had shorter stays than non-whites.

The larger the hospital, the longer the average length of stay. A voluntary hospital episode was associated with the longest, and a proprietary hospital the shortest length of stay.

NCHS

1973   *Utilization of Short-Stay Hospitals — Summary of Nonmedical Statistics: United States-1970.* Series 13. Number 14.

This report presents statistics on the utilization of short-stay hospitals from the 1970 Hospital Discharge Survey.

The report is in two sections — one by detailed ages of patients under 15 years of age and the other by four broad age categories. Discharges, days of care, and average length of stay are reported by age, sex and color of the discharged patients and by geographic region, bed size, and type of ownership of the hospitals.

Of an estimated 3.9 million discharged patients under 15 years of age, the proportion of males was about twice that of females, and rates of discharge decreased as age increased. The youngest group had the longest length of stay. White patients used proportionately fewer days of care than nonwhites.

For those under 15 years of age, the North Central Region had 2½ times the number of discharges as the West and the latter had the shortest average length of stay. As the size of the hospital increased, the relative percent of those under one year of age increased. Regardless of the type of hospital ownership, patients under 15 used fewer days of care than others.

In 1970 the discharge rate for males 65 years and over was about four times and the days of care rate 11 times the rates for patients less than 15. Among females 65 and over the rates were even higher. White patients in a single age group over 15 used less than their proportionate share of days of care and nonwhites more.

The biggest difference in average length of stay between regions for those over 15 years of age was found between those of the Northeast and West, the latter having the shortest average length of stay of any region. As age and hospital size increased, the average length of stay increased. There were significant differences in the distribution of patients 15-64 years of age in hospitals by type of ownership.

Newman, J. and O.W. Anderson

1972   *Patterns of Dental Services Utilization in the United States: A Nationwide Social Survey.* Research Series No. 30. Chicago: Center for Health Administration Studies, University of Chicago.

The purpose of this study is to report the findings from a nationwide survey of dental service utilization.

Early in 1965 the staff of the National Opinion Research Center (NORC) interviewed a national sample of households to obtain data concerning the use of dental services for the calendar year 1964. In all, 3,165 families were interviewed.

Utilization rates were reported in terms of expenditures and mean visits per family (or person), the proportion of families (or individuals) with visits and the type of service utilized. The issue of the continuity of dental care was also considered.

The variables for which the utilization rates were examined were age, sex, race, education of head of household, occupation of head of household, family life cycle, family size, family income, ability to pay $500 dental bill, prior income level, region, residence, population per dentist, dental symptoms, and tartar on teeth.

Cross-tabulations and AID were used to analyze the data.

Age, race, education and occupation of the head of the household, income and dental health status were the most crucial variables for understanding dental utilization. Other variables such as sex, region, residence, population per dentist, family life cycle and family size were less important. Despite large increases in the proportion of persons with dental visits since the thirties, dental use remained low relative to other health services. Nonwhites seemed to have the least continuous dental care, based on when dental care was last received.

Noble, J.H., et al.

1971 "Variations in visits to hospital emergency care facilities: ritualistic and meteorological factors affecting supply and demand." *Med. Care* 9 (September-October): 415-427.

The purpose of this study is to determine the relationship between days of the week, holiday travel, and meteorological patterns on emergency unit visits, traffic accident injuries and "sick assist" cases served by ambulances of the Boston Police Department.

Data were collected from the emergency units of Beth Israel Hospital, Peter Bent Brigham Hospital and Children's Hospital Medical Center and from Boston Police Department Records for 1968.

The utilization indices examined included emergency visits to hospital by mode of transportation (police or private ambulance), traffic accident ambulance runs and "sick assist" runs by the Boston Police Department ambulances.

The various indices for which the utilization variables were examined included the days of the week, whether it was a holiday or day on which pre- or post-holiday travel occurs, and an index of weather conditions.

Stepwise regression was used to analyze the data.

The authors conclude that differences in the distribution of injuries vs. disease and emergent vs. nonurgent conditions may be reduced to variations in levels of risk attributable to the weather and holiday traffic. Though the patterns vary somewhat in each hospital, for all three hospitals there was a tendency for traffic, other than ambulances, to increase during favorable weather.

Nyman, K. and E. Kalimo

> 1973   "National sickness insurance and the use of physi-
>   cians' services in Finland." *Soc. Sci. Med.* 7 (July):
>   541-553.

This study evaluates the effects of the introduction of national sickness insurance in Finland (1964) on the use of services.

Household surveys of the non-institutionalized population of Finland
were conducted during May-June, 1964, prior to the introduction of
national sickness insurance, and in May-June, 1968, after it had been in
operation several years.

The utilization index reported was the number of consultations with a
physician per 100 adults per 100 days in the survey year.

Information was collected on the number of local physicians per
10,000 inhabitants and the age, sex, income, region, residence, distance
to the nearest physician and number of sickness days experienced by
respondents.

Cross-tabulation of rates and AID analysis were used to analyze the
data.

National sickness insurance seemed to have increased use, particularly among the acutely ill of the low-income. Men apparently seek care
in smaller numbers than women when disease is mild, but at more severe
stages of illness, men end up using more services than women. The
number of consultations with physicians decreased in all categories of
sickness days, with increasing remoteness of residence and with de-
creasing density of physicians in the locality. National sickness insurance apparently did not have a marked effect on the distribution of
physicians, however.

Olendzki, M.C., et al.

> 1972   "The impact of Medicaid on private care for the
>   urban poor." *Med. Care* 10 (May-June): 201-206.

This study investigates the extent to which Medicaid opened up
private medical care for the urban poor.

Former welfare clients in New York City (n=729), were interviewed
on five interview waves — three before Medicaid (1961-62, 1962-63,
1963-64) and the two after (1968-69, 1969-70).

Information on the respondents' utilization was obtained from a question about the "main place" they received medical care. Consumer
satisfaction was reflected in responses to a question whether they would

prefer to go to a hospital clinic or emergency room, or to a private doctor, if it didn't cost them anything and they could choose; the reasons for using a clinic or emergency room while preferring a private doctor, and respondents' impression of how many local doctors accepted Medicaid patients.

Responses to these questions were sought before and after the introduction of Medicaid.

The proportion who considered a private doctor their "main place" for medical care rose from one percent before Medicaid to ten percent afterwards. The large majority continued to use clinics. Some who preferred private care were unable to take advantage of it because of practical barriers (private care too expensive, due to New York State Medicaid cutbacks; special facilities or treatment were needed, etc.), but many others claimed to prefer clinic care. Those who preferred clinics may be divided into two groups: 1) those who had positive and sensible reasons, such as the "facilities were better" or the "doctors more competent," and 2) those for whom private care seemed beyond the range of "accessible" alternatives.

Palmore, E. and C. Luikart

1972   "Health and social factors related to life satisfaction." *J. Health Soc. Behav.* 13 (March): 68-80.

This study analyzes the impact of health, activity, social-psychological and socio-economic variables on a measure of life satisfaction.

Data for this analysis came from the Duke University Adaptation Study, an interdisciplinary longitudinal study of 502 persons aged 45-69 at the beginning of the study in 1968.

Life satisfaction was measured by the "Cantril Ladder." The respondent was presented with a picture of a ladder and was asked if the top of the nine-rung ladder represented the best possible life and the bottom the worst, where he would rank himself at the present time.

Satisfaction was correlated with the health (self-rated health, performance status), activity (organizational activity, social activity hours, production hours, social contacts, employment), social-psychological characteristics (internal control, career anchorage, confidence, marital status, sexual enjoyment, moves, intelligence), socio-economic status (income, education age, sex) of the respondents.

Zero-order and multiple correlation coefficient were used to analyze the data.

Self-rated health was found to be most highly correlated with life satisfaction. The amount of organizational activity and belief in internal control were the second and third most important variables related to life satisfaction. Organizational activity, in turn, was mainly related to intelligence and to internal control orientation among the men, but among women it was mainly related to lack of employment and to physical performance status. Several variables thought to be related to life satisfaction were found to have little or no relationship: age, sex, total social contacts, career anchorage, marital status, and intelligence.

Pettengill, J.H.

1972   "Trends in hospital use by the aged." *Soc. Sec. Bull.* 35 (July): 3-15.

This article compares data from a variety of sources on the hospital utilization experience of persons aged 65 and over during the period 1963-1971.

Data used in this paper are derived from seven sources — National Center for Health Statistics Health Interview Survey (HIS), National Center for Health Statistics Hospital Discharge Survey (HDS), Columbia University Survey (CUS) on the early impact of Medicare, American Hospital Association Hospital Indicators Study, American Hospital Association *Guide Issue,* Social Security Administration Current Medical Survey (CMS) and Social Security Administration Medicare Control Records (MCR).

Information was reported on the numbers of discharges and stays per 1,000 days of care per 1,000 and average lengths of stay.

The changes over the years prior to and after the introduction of Medicare are reported.

Cross-tabulation of rates are used to summarize the findings.

In the first three years following the inception of Medicare, use of hospital services by the aged increased at an annual rate of six to thirteen percent. Since 1969, however, hospital utilization by this age group has been declining one to three percent annually, mostly as a result of a decline in average length of stay. Comparison with similar data for persons under age 65 reveals that a significant redistribution of hospital care between the age group and those aged 65 and over has occurred since 1965. It is likely that aged persons increased their use of hospital services to some extent at the expense of persons under 65.

Phelps, C.E. and J.P. Newhouse

1972 "Effect of coinsurance: a multivariate analysis." *Soc. Sec. Bull.* 35 (June): 20-28; 44.

This study uses multiple regression analysis to study the impact of coinsurance on physician visits, physician expense, ancillary services and ancillary services expense in a comprehensive, prepaid group practice plan.

Data were collected from the Stanford University Group Health Plan (GHP), available to employees there.

The dependent variables considered were physician visits, physician expense, ancillary service use and ancillary service expense.

For each person, the following data were also available: age, sex, relation to subscriber, distance from the Medical Center, occupational status and family size.

Multiple regression analysis was used to analyze the data.

When a 25-percent coinsurance rate was introduced, the members' demand for medical care was significantly reduced — holding all other variables (age, sex, distance, etc.) constant.

Purola, T.

1973 *Health Insurance, the Incidence of Illness, and the Use of Medical Services.* Unpub. manuscript. Helsinki: Research Institute for Social Security.

The purpose of this study is to report on the effectiveness of a national sickness insurance scheme introduced in Finland in 1964.

Data came from a 1968 follow-up survey of the Finnish population. An earlier study was conducted in 1964 prior to the introduction of the national sickness insurance program.

Information is reported on physician use and illness (chronic illness, sick days, bed days, diagnoses) by age, sex, region and place of residence in Finland.

Cross-tabulation of distributions and t-test of statistical significance are used to analyze the data.

The author discusses a framework for the study, that includes the social psychological predispositions and processes that lead individuals to seek care and the economic and system-relevant resources that enable them to procure such services. A basic hypothesis tested is that the introduction of universal sickness insurance coverage effectively lowers the cost of treatment for the sick. The use of services subsequently becomes independent of income; and is determined in accordance with the incidence of illness.

The results of the study do not confirm that universal insurance coverage was as successful as expected in reducing the barriers to the seeking of needed medical care. The low-income and those persons in areas of low medical resource availability are still at a disadvantage with respect to getting care when the need arises. The author concludes that, in addition to national sickness insurance, which is primarily a financing mechanism, attention should be directed to the organization of the medical care system itself and to the introduction of programs to enhance the consumer's willingness to seek care when symptoms are experienced.

Rabin, D.L. (ed.)

> 1972   "International comparisons of medical care." *Milb. Mem. Fund Quart.* 50 (July): 1-99.

This paper reports the organization and some preliminary findings of the World Health Organization International Collaborative Study of Medical Care Utilization (WHO/ICS-MCU).

Household interviews were conducted in samples from Canada (Grande Prairie, Saskatchewan, Fraser and Jersey); United States (Northwestern Vermont, Baltimore); Argentina (Buenos Aires), United Kingdom (Liverpool); Finland (Helsinki); Poland (Lodz); and Yugoslavia (Banat, Rijeka) during the months from June 1, 1968 to May 31, 1969.

Utilization indices reported are the use of physicians and other health workers within two weeks, use of dentists within one month, use of hospitals within one year, use of prescribed and nonprescribed medicines within two days and reasons for the most recent physician and dentist visit.

Information collected on the health delivery system included its resources — ratios of physicians and number of hours available per 10,000 population, ratio of dentists, nurses and other health workers per 10,000 population, and short- and long-term hospital beds per 1,000 population — and organization— system points of entry, distributional responsibility, administrative requirements, drug dispersing policies, health indicators, public health indices, economic indices and systems description.

The designers of the study posited a model of predisposing, enabling and need components that were said to explain utilization behavior. The predisposing variables included age, sex, marital status, family size, personal attitudes, anxiety and smoking habits. The enabling variables were said to be income, health insurance coverage, educational level, identification of personal physician, ability to meet unusual expenses and travel time to the nearest doctor. Need included indices of both acute and chronic conditions. "Acute" need was reflected in bed days and restricted activity days in two weeks, departure from health and perceived severity, and dental morbidity one month prior to the interview. "Chronic" need was gauged by the reported presence of a chronic disease, an impairment or unusual defect and the presence of symptoms indicating angina pectoris, rheumatoid arthritis, breathlessness or chronic bronchitis.

Cross-tabulation of percentage distributions and path analysis were used to analyze the data.

The model for this study contains many of the elements necessary for a framework for the study of access, also — characteristics of the health services system (resource ratios and system characteristics) — and the population-at-risk (predisposing, enabling and need) that determine utilization.

This publication includes background and methodological sections on the organizational development of the surveys, the methods used in conducting them and some results of reliability and validity studies of the data.

Other studies on the ecologic, system-relevant and behavioral results of the surveys show that the model used in this study is borne out for the different regions. Differences in utilization, according to these preliminary analyses, were attributable to differences in the properties of the delivery system and the populations in the respective areas.

Richardson, J.D. and F.D. Scutchfield

> 1973   "Priorities in health care: the consumer's viewpoint in an Appalachian community." *Amer. J. Public Health* 63 (January): 79-82.

This study was made to determine consumer attitudes toward health needs in an Appalachian community, and to find out what are the priorities of such consumers for care.

Data were provided from a random household survey in Rowan County, Kentucky in May, 1970.

Consumer attitudes on what constituted the major problems of health care delivery in their area were reported.

Attitudes were compared for the rural and urban populations in the sample.

Cross-tabulation of percentage distributions were used to analyze the data.

The major area of concern was the high cost of care, followed by the lack of physician availability and specialty services. These priorities were, in general, true for both the rural and urban sub-populations.

Richardson, W.C.

> 1971   *Ambulatory Use of Physician's Services in Re-*
> *sponse to Illness Episodes in a Low-Income Neigh-*
> *borhood.* Research Series No. 29. Chicago: Center
> for Health Administration Studies, University of
> Chicago.

This study identifies factors that are related to the individual and his environment, poverty among them, which influence his response behavior when he becomes sick.

Household interviews were conducted in the Red Hook section of Brooklyn, New York, one of several low-income target areas chosen for the introduction of neighborhood health centers sponsored by the Office of Economic Opportunity.

The utilization indices reported included the delay before seeing a doctor (in days); whether there was an initial physician contact or not, the number of revisits; and the total amounts of care received, in response to an illness episode.

Information was also collected on the perceived seriousness of the illness episode, the race-ethnicity of the respondent, education of family head, adjusted current income, third-party coverage, bed-disability days experienced, usual source of care, and physician-rated seriousness of the condition, and the person's usual activity (wage earner, housewife, child).

Regression analysis, using the Tobit model to correct for skewness in the distribution of the dependent variable, was the mode of analysis employed.

The author reports the effect of the various socioeconomic, source of care and illness variables on the level of delay, whether or not there was an initial contact and the number of revisits for a given episode of illness. He further emphasizes the importance of using an episodic approach to delimit *patterns* of care-seeking in response to illness.

Robertson, R.L.

1972   "Comparative medical care use under prepaid group
practice and free choice plans: a case study."
Inquiry 9 (September): 70-76.

The purpose of this study was to compare the utilization experiences
of a blue plan and group practice-type insurance scheme.

Data were collected from medical records of public school teachers
covered by a prepaid group practice plan with comprehensive benefits
and teachers in the same community subscribing to an extensive non-
group insurance plan.

Utilization was reported for inpatient admission rates — medical and
surgical admissions, patient days and outpatient physician contacts for
medical cases.

The two plans were compared and a t-test used to evaluate the
statistical significance to the differences between the plans.

The group practice plan, in contrast to the blue plan, had lower
medical and surgical inpatient admissions, fewer hospital days and a
higher rate of outpatient physician contacts for medical cases.

Satin, D.G.

1973   " 'Help': The hospital emergency unit patient and
his presenting picture." *Med. Care* 11 (July-
August): 328-337.

The purpose of this study is to see how the illness behavior of the
emergency room user is influenced by his socio-cultural and social
psychological background.

A random sample (n=257) of applicants to the emergency unit (EU) of
an urban general hospital were selected to be interviewed by research
psychiatrist interviewers.

The distribution of the physical and psychological complaints of
emergency room users were reported.

The effects of age, the number of generations in the United States,
socio-economic status, usual source of care, emotional stress and severity of stress on the nature of the presenting complaint were analyzed.

Multiple regression and correlation analysis were used to report the
findings.

The presenting picture of the EU user is described as manifesting a
broad range of needs and non-illness-related influences. Covert
recent life stress was a major predictor of the presenting picture. The

EU applicant, was more apt to be nonwhite or a recent immigrant, have no regular source of care, unemployed and in the lowest socio-economic class. The author urges more attention be given to the social-emotional background of the hospital emergency unit users in the interest of improving the delivery of emergency medical care.

Satin, D.G. and F.J. Duhl

1972   "Help?: the hospital emergency unit as community physician." *Med. Care* 10 (May-June): 248-260.

This study presents data on the prior treatment experience of patients coming to the hospital emergency room, their paths to the facility, the varying interpretations of the health problems found, administrative and medical management and final disposition.

A random sample (n=257) of applicants to the emergency unit (EU) of an urban general hospital were selected to be interviewed by research psychiatrist interviewers.

The nature of the presenting problem, its severity, duration, the source of referral, the attending clinic service and disposition of the complaint are reported.

A Chi-square test of significance and Cramer's V were used to analyze the relationship of these components of an individual's visit to the EU.

The authors point out that the hospital emergency unit is increasingly becoming a center for the receipt of ambulatory medical care. They suggest that the patient's and physician's definitions of the presenting problem of the EU user may differ. The emergency unit staff, especially, may fail to deal with the psychiatric and social problems brought by the patient.

Evidence that patients tend to view the emergency room as a primary care source is reflected in the findings that over 80 percent of EU users lived nearby, for half it is the first source applied to, three quarters had not been treated previously, one quarter were treated by the triage physician only, for one quarter no referrals for treatment elsewhere were made, and more than half the sample came on their own initially or were referred by family or friends, rather than medical professionals.

Schoen, M.H.

1973   "Observation of selected dental services under two prepayment mechanisms." *Amer. J. Public Health* 63 (August): 727-731.

The purpose of this study is to compare the dental utilization experience of a prepaid group practice and open panel fee-for-service plan.

Data were collected from patient charts at the group practice offices and from claim forms at the California Dental Service (CDS) Insurance Company for members of Warehousemen's Union Local 26 in Los Angeles for the years 1963-1966.

The indices of utilization examined were as follows: utilization of one or more dental services, prophylaxes, permanent teeth extracted, root canal fillings, number of units of crown and bridgework provided, number of partial and full dentures constructed.

Utilization rates for the group practice and open panel plans were compared over a three-year period.

Histograms and cross-tabulation of percentage distributions were used to reporting the findings.

The group practice plan had higher utilization rates, prophylaxis and removable prosthetic rates. Extraction rates and crowns and bridge rates were similar. Root canal therapy was performed too infrequently to be meaningful. Assuming the socio-economic level of the population to be average, the group practice plan clearly achieved better dental care behavior than is true nationally.

Schneider, G.E. and S. Fox

    1973   "Health care coverage and out-of-pocket expenditures of Detroit families." *Inquiry* 10 (December): 49-57.

The purpose of this study was to investigate the demographic characteristics and out-of-pocket health expenditures of Detroit families covered by various types of health insurance.

A random sample of 5,970 families living in Detroit provided the data. The study was conducted from September, 1971, through August, 1972, by the Detroit team of the Michigan Health Survey (funded by grants from the Michigan Association of Regional Medical Programs and the Michigan Office of Comprehensive Health Planning).

Information on the type of health insurance coverage and percent distributions of out-of-pocket expenditures were reported by race, family size, family income, and education of head of household.

Cross-tabulation of percent distributions and charts were used to summarize the findings.

Both Blue Cross and Blue Shield and commercial insurance companies were found to be insuring the middle- and upper middle-class segments of the population. Of families with incomes under $4,000, Blue Cross and Blue Shield were covering, or helping to cover, 29 percent of these low-income families, while all commercial insurance companies combined were covering only about 7 percent of these families. About 28 percent of all families paid out-of-pocket expenditures of approximately $7 for drugs in the month for which data were collected. About 17 percent of the Blue Cross and Blue Shield families had approximately $14 for preventive care. Four percent (4%) of these families paid approximately $27 for eyeglasses. Twenty percent (20%) of the Blue Cross and Blue Shield spent money on dental care compared to 12 percent of the commercial insurance families.

Scitovsky, A.A. and N.M. Snyder

> 1972   "Effect of coinsurance on use of physician ser-
>   vices." *Soc. Sec. Bull.* 35 (June): 3-19.

This study is concerned with the impact of the introduction of a 25-percent coinsurance provision on the demand for physician services under a comprehensive prepaid plan of medical care.

The data are from the Group Health Plan (GHP), offered since 1965 by Stanford University to all its employees who work at least 50 percent of full-time. It provides almost complete medical care in and out of the hospital for employees and their dependents.

Information on the per capita number and per capita cost of physician visits and outpatient ancillary services by type and site of service and reported.

Utilization and cost data are reported prior to and after the introduction of the coinsurance mechanism, controlling for age, sex, occupational and insurance coverage status.

Cross-tabulation of rates are used to report the findings.

The findings suggest that the coinsurance provision led to a substantial decline in the demand for services. The per capita number of all physician services went down 24.1 percent and per capita cost 23.8 percent. Physician hospital services declined least and home health visits most. There were few clearly discernible patterns of change that could be attributed to demographic characteristics, such as age, sex, occupation or insurance status.

Shannon, G.W., et al.

> 1973   "Time and distance: the journey for medical care."
>   *Intl. J. Health Services,* 3 (Spring): 237-243.

This study demonstrates the differences in conclusions that can be reached regarding the relative accessibility of health facilities as a result of using travel time as opposed to linear distance as the independent variable.

A sample of adult residents from the metropolitan area of Cleveland, Ohio, was interviewed in the fall of 1967 to get information for the study.

Contact with a health practitioner or facility — doctor, dentist, or hospital — constituted the utilization index.

Information was also collected on the distance each individual must travel for each health service, the time spent in travel, the distance of the individual's residence from the central business district for each individual and the average speed of travel to the health facility.

Correlation and regression analysis were used to analyze the data.

The authors conclude that "considering travel time and linear distance independently of each other as measures of accessibility of health care facilities produce different results." There is no consistent relationship between the distance of one's residence from the central business district and travel time, because of intervening variables such as the average speed traveled.

Shortell, S.

1972   *A Model of Physician Referral Behavior: A Test of Exchange Theory in Medical Practice.* Research Series No. 31. Chicago: Center for Health Administration Studies, University of Chicago.

The purpose of this study is to analyze the professional relationships which underlie the delivery of medical care, especially physician referral behavior.

Internists in the northern suburbs of Chicago were the study population. Data collection instruments included a survey questionnaire and a set of referral verification forms on which physicians were asked to log information on referred patients over a two-week period, May 7-21, 1971.

Rates of referral examined for each practice were as follows:

$$\text{inflow rate} = \frac{\text{number of patients received on referral from other physicians}}{\text{total number of patient visits for a given week of practice}}$$

$$\text{outflow rate} = \frac{\text{number of patients referred to other physicians}}{\text{total number of patient visits for a given week of practice}}$$

$$\text{agency rate} = \frac{\text{number of patients referred to health agencies (excluding hospital admissions)}}{\text{total number of patient visits for a given week of practice}}$$

Information was also collected on the patterns of referrals — who refers to whom in terms of status, friendship, hospital appointments, distance between offices, reciprocity of relationship, etc.

Data on selected physician characteristics, e.g., organization and volume of practice, years in practice, caseload severity, professional competence, whether or not he is board-certified, whether or not he has published professional articles, his overall professional status, and his satisfaction with referrals were also collected.

Regression analysis and sociometric matrices were used to analyze the data.

Using exchange theory as a model, the author advances and tests a series of hypotheses relating the characteristics of physicians and their practices to the rate and patterns of their referrals to other physicians or agencies. The author traces, in some detail, the importance of professional status and other characteristics on the inflow, outflow, and agency referral rates for internists with subspecialties and those who are generalists. The physicians' satisfaction with their referral outcomes are described, as are the patterns of referral themselves (status of physicians involved in exchange, primary hospital appointments of physicians, friendship patterns, etc.)

Also, see S. Shortell and O.W. Anderson, "The physician referral process: a theoretical perspective." Health Services Research 6 (Spring): 39-48.

Shortell, S.

1973   "Patterns of medical care: issues of access, cost, and continuity." Paper presented at Workshop, Center for Health Administration Studies, University of Chicago (April 5).

This article treats the access concept *per se* and develops some indicators of the continuity of care.

Data are presented from the CHAS-NORC 1971 survey of health services utilization on those women who experienced a pregnancy during a survey year.

The dimensions of utilization examined to reflect continuity were as follows: total sources of care, total physician visits and visits per source for woman with a past pregnancy, and the reason woman went to a designated source — usual doctc˜ or clinic, referred by usual doctor, etc.

The preceding use measures were analyzed by the race, education, family income, insurance coverage, regular source of care and residence of the respondent.

Cross-tabulation of percentage distributions were used to analyze the data.

The higher income, whites as opposed to nonwhites, the better-educated, and those with insurance, had greater access-continuity, according to Shortell's indices. Those reporting a clinic as their regular source of care had less access than those reporting the use of particular physicians. In general, women receiving care from board-certified physicians experienced greater access than those whose attending physicians were not board-certified.

The author points out that several criteria of access appear in the literature — cost; geographic or temporal availability; internal economy of staffing, waiting time, etc.; psychological dimensions of fear, etc.; and knowledge. He suggests, however, that there must be some external validation of these criteria, by examining utilization rates for different groups who possess these attributes.

Simon, J.L. and D.B. Smith

> 1973   "Change in location of a student health service: a quasi-experimental evaluation of the effects of distance on utilization." *Med. Care* 11 (January-February): 59-67.

This study analyzes the impact of the relocation of a student health center on students' use of the facility.

Data were collected from clinic records of the University of Rochester Student Health Service before and after it was moved off-campus.

The average number of visits per student each month in the years immediately prior to (1965-66, 1966-67) and after (1967-68, 1968-69) the change in location, were analyzed.

The number of visits were considered in the context of the nature of the presenting complaint.

Graphs, a Chi-square test of significance and partial correlation coefficients were used to analyze the data.

The results showed a significant reduction in the number of visits to the clinic after it was moved, that could not be accounted for by a trend over time. No appreciable changes occurred in an infirmary, whose location remained unchanged. Utilization for respiratory complaints and immunizations seemed to be more affected by the move than were more specialized services.

Solon, J.A. and R.D. Rigg

1972   "Patterns of medical care among users of hospital emergency units." *Med. Care* 10 (January-February): 60-72.

This study attempts to document the overall pattern of medical care, from all sources, of emergency room users.

All users of the emergency room facilities of two hospitals for a one-week period constituted the sample. One of the hospitals was an inner-city hospital with a substantial lower-income population and the other a suburban hospital with a predominantly middle-class population.

Utilization information was reported on the number of individuals who used the emergency rooms of the two hospitals during the study period and the purpose of the visit; the central source of medical care of the individuals and how often this source is used; and other sources of care and how often each source is used.

The social class and income of the users was reported.

Cross tabulation of percentage distributions were used to analyze the data.

Eighty-five percent (85%) of the suburban hospital users see a private physician as their central source of care. Only 59 percent of the inner city hospital emergency room users had a physician as a usual source of care. The outpatient department was the central source of care for 20 percent of the inner city population. The emergency room was used by both groups mainly for emergencies and did not play a large role in their overall configuration of health care. Only fourteen percent (14%) of the inner-city residents and seven percent (7%) of suburban residents used the emergency room as their prime source of care.

Solon, J.A., et al.

1967   "Delineating episodes of medical care." *Amer. J. Public Health* 57 (March): 401-408.

This study points out the usefulness of considering an episode of illness in measuring utilization.

It deals with data collected on the medical care received by nursing students during their three years in a hospital-based school.

Solon defines an episode of medical care as follows:

An episode of medical care is a block of one or more medical services received by an individual during a period of relatively continuous contact with one or more providers of service, in relation to a particular medical problem or situation.

A medical care episode includes: (1) the patient's medical problem or situation, (2) the time intervals between services, and (3) the nature of the medical management.

An episode of medical care is presented in the context of the diagnostic category or presenting complaint of a selected sample of nursing students.

The authors conclude that observing an episode of medical care is a better means to reflect the pattern and continuity of care-seeking.

Somers, A.R.

1971   *Health Care in Transition: Directions for the Future.* Chicago: Hospital Research and Educational Trust.

This book is a comprehensive treatment of the range of problems that comprise the health care crisis in the United States.

It is a conceptual rather than an empirical article.

This book points up the paradoxes that characterize the medical care crisis with respect to the physician, the patient, the hospital and recent developments in financing, and then offers some goals and guidelines for dealing with this crisis.

With respect to physicians, the author argues:

A considerable part of the problem . . . is the fact that so many people still lack access to good health care. For many it is quantitatively deficient. For many more, including many in middle-income and upper-income categories, it is qualitatively lacking, particu-

larly in the educational influence of a good doctor-patient relationship, a lack that probably disturbs the patient even more than it
does the doctor (p. 23).

Regarding the hospital, she points up that increasing use of emergency
rooms is not due to increases in emergency cases or traumas, necessarily, but because of a "demand for instant care at the convenience of both
physician and patient." She also describes the problems of physician-
administrator conflict and some of the factors that account for varying
hospital utilization rates by region — such as the degree of urbanization,
differences in per capita income, differences in number of doctors and
hospital beds, extent to which care for chronic illness is provided, etc.

Shortcomings in current financing programs — gaps and duplications,
etc. — and rising provider costs have created problems — inability to
provide comprehensive coverage and continuing dissatisfaction on the
part of providers and consumers.

The author concludes by offering several solutions to the difficulties
described — a national program of consumer education, redefinition of
professional roles to assure personal care, rationalization of community
health services and the role of the hospitals, and national health insurance.

Sparer, G. and A. Anderson

    1973   "Utilization and cost experience of low-income
              families in four prepaid group-practice plans." *New
              Eng. J. Med.* 289 (July 12): 67-72.

This study compares use rates for low-income families in several
group practice plan settings.

Records of regular plan members and OEO enrollees in four group
practice plans — Kaiser (Fontana, California); Kaiser (Portland,
Oregon); Group Health of Puget Sound (Washington); Health Insurance Plan of New York (Suffolk Co.) — provided the data.

Utilization rates by service (physician, nonphysician, laboratory,
x-ray, prescriptions, home health), physician encounter rates per 1,000
persons, hospital admissions, length of stay and expenditures, comprised the utilization indices.

The four plans were described in terms of their age distributions, their
average family size, number of families and number of members in the
plan.

Cross-tabulations of rates and percentages were used to report the
findings.

The low-income families, enrolled in the group practice plans through arrangements supported by the Office of Economic Opportunity (OEO), required six months to achieve a utilization level not exceeding that of the regular plan members. Compared to national data, costs were less because of reductions in hospital days for the poor under pre-paid group practice arrangements. The number of inpatient days per 100 OEO enrollees was 600 days under the group plan. The national average for low-income people under the age of 65 is about 1,000 days.

Steele, J.L. and W.H. McBroom

    1972   "Conceptual and empirical dimensions of health behavior." *J. Health Soc. Behav.* 13 (December): 382-392.

The purpose of this study is to empirically investigate the meaning and nature of the concept "health behavior."

A multi-staged random sample of 3,243 individuals from almost 1,000 households, representing a three percent sample of a large rural area of Montana were interviewed to provide the data.

Four indicators of health behavior used were: 1) evidence of having physical checkups over period of twelve months; 2) evidence of having eye visit in past twelve months; 3) evidence of having a dental visit in past twelve months; and 4) evidence of having insurance in past twelve months. The first three types of health behavior were trichotomized according to whether the person said he had the checkup when he did *not* feel ill, had it for other reasons or did not have a checkup. The insurance variable was trichotomized according to whether the person reported having both medical and hospital insurance, had less comprehensive coverage, or reported no insurance coverage.

A socio-economic status (SES) index was constructed on the basis of family income, occupation and education of the dominant female in the household.

Frequency distributions and gamma correlations between the indicators were used to analyze the data.

The health behavior index or indicator chosen makes a great difference in whether an SES group is high or low in health behavior. If only those who had a checkup for non-illness-related reasons are considered in constructing a "health behavior" index, 80 to 90 percent of the sample may be said not to practice health behavior. If those who sought a checkup for *any* reason are considered, the percent is much smaller.

Teller, C.H.

1973   "Access to medical care of migrants in a Honduran
            City." *J. Health Soc. Behav.* 14 (September):
            214-226.

This study tests the hypothesis that the traditional cultural attitudes
and beliefs of the internal migrants in Latin American cities explain their
reluctance to make use of modern scientific medical care.

Data were collected from a sample of a low-income quadrant of the
city of San Pedro Sula, Honduras, during late 1970 and early 1971.
Migration and health questionnaires, retrospective life histories, clinical
exams, and participant observation comprised the data collection
mechanisms.

Utilization was reported in terms of 1) access to professionals —
utilization of a licensed medical practitioner or utilization of the private
or public sector in the preceding two weeks, and 2) treatment in a private
system through consultations with non-professionals when ill or the use
of household remedies and other forms of self-care when ill in the two
weeks preceding the interview.

A behavioral model of health service use was introduced to explain
utilization. The predisposing factors included the age and sex distribution of the family and its migration status — communities of origin,
intermediate communities and time in the city. Enabling variables referred to the socio-economic status of respondents (education, occupation,
income and prestige) and their system orientation (health insurance,
discontent). Need or health status was reflected in illness and symptoms
reported by respondents.

Percentage distributions and histograms were used to portray the
data.

Findings showed low access rates of the population to professional
medical care institutions. No consistent relationships were found between migratory status and access to medical care when socio-economic
status was held constant. Positive selectivity, prior urban experience,
and extensive kinship networks aided most migrants in the transition to
urban life. Whether a person or family manifested modern medical care
utilization behavior depended more on the urban opportunity structure
than on traditional cultural beliefs and attitudes.

Torrens, P.R. and D.G. Yedvab

1970   "Variations among emergency room populations: a

comparison of four hospitals in New York City."
Med. Care 8 (January-February): 60-75.

The purpose of this study was to determine the importance of urban hospital emergency rooms as a source of general medical care.

Four hospitals, located in four different sections of New York City, and representing a cross-section of hospitals in the city were selected for study. A sample of 1,113 patient-users of the emergency rooms in each hospital were interviewed.

The rate and purpose of using the hospital emergency room in each hospital was reported.

Characteristics of the population of users was described in terms of their socio-economic status, presenting complaint, level of government financial assistance and insurance coverage, prescriptions issued for the patient and recommended follow-up care, and the most frequently utilized sources of medical care during the previous year.

Cross-tabulation of percentage distributions were used to analyze the data.

After studying four different emergency rooms which serve four different urban neighborhoods, the authors conclude that there is no standard model that describes the emergency room. The results of the study suggest that the role the emergency room assumes is shaped by the particular needs of the people served and by the willingness of the hospital to adapt to these needs. The authors list three general roles for the emergency room, that may be found to some degree in any emergency room: 1) trauma-treatment center; 2) private physician and outpatient department substitute in off-hours; and 3) family physician for the urban poor. By assessing what types of populations the hospital serves and what particular needs the residents will seek to fulfill through the emergency room, hospital administrators can better design their emergency rooms to meet these demands.

U.S. Department of Agriculture

1973   *Health Services in Rural America.* Agriculture Information Bulletin No. 362. Washington: U.S. Department of Agriculture, Rural Development Service.

This paper points out some of the problems of health care delivery in rural areas.

Data from the National Center for Health Statistics, the American Medical Association, the American Hospital Association, etc. are summarized.

Utilization data on the number of physician visits per person per year, visits per 100 families to selected medical specialists and practitioners per year, number of dental visits per person per year and the number of persons hospitalized per 1,000 population per year are reported.

Characteristics of the health delivery system in rural areas, especially the availability of resources — physicians and other medical practitioners per 100,000 population and hospital beds per 100,000 population — are described, as are the characteristics of the rural population itself, in terms of their age; race; family income; insurance coverage; place of residence; restricted activity days and major activity limitation due to chronic illness; and the number of dental needs per patient.

Cross-tabulation of percentage distributions are used to report the findings.

The authors report: "One must conclude that rural and urban people do not have equal access to health care services. Rural areas are deficient in professional medical personnel, physical health care facilities, and the ability to afford the financial costs of illnesses." As a result, the rates of utilization of health services continue to be lower and the need for care greater in rural areas.

vanDyke, F. and V. Brown

    1972   "Organized home care: an alternative to institutions." *Inquiry* 9 (June): 3-16.

This study was an evaluation of patients receiving services from Medicare-certified home-health agencies, to explore the barriers to more and better utilization of organized health-related home care.

Data were obtained from 275 patients who were receiving home-health care under a specific agency in one of the nine counties of New York City, Long Island and Westchester, New York. Physicians and public health nurses collected the data, which included reports of physical examinations and open-ended interviews with the patients.

The utilization patterns of home-care recipients were examined.

The demographic characteristics (age, chronic limitation) and barriers to c:·e (insurance, income) of the users of home-care services were analyzed.

Cross-tabulation of percent distributions were used to summarize the findings.

The authors concluded that home-health care was a valuable and viable alternative to long-term institutional care, but that there is a need to expand and coordinate such services, to rationalize delivery and to make this care available as a health insurance benefit. The home-health care population was predominantly 65 or older and most were chronically ill or permanently disabled. In order to remain at home, rather than in an institution, home-health care, funded under health insurance programs, must be made available to them.

Weinerman, E.R., et al.

1966   "Yale studies in ambulatory medical care. V. Determinants of hospital emergency services." *Amer. J. Public Health* 56 (July): 1037-1056.

The purpose of this study is to delineate the demographic characteristics of the emergency room population, to identify the usual patterns of seeking and receiving medical care, and to assess the major factors affecting the urgency of need for such care.

A sample of 2,028 visits to the emergency room (ER) of Yale-New Haven Hospital, during the two-week period from July 9 to July 22, 1964 was taken.

Persons who visited the emergency room were described in terms of their age, sex, marital status, minority group status, location of residence, duration of residence in city, length of time at current address, employment, occupation, educational level, social class, usual source of medical care, previous medical care, duration of current disorder and urgency evaluation by medical staff.

Cross-tabulation of percentage distributions, graphs, a Chi-square test of statistical significance and a multivariate analysis technique for qualitative data were the modes of analysis employed.

The emergency room population, compared to the total population, had more children and young adults, more males, more non-married, more nonwhites, and more inner city residents. The general population and emergency room population were quite similar in their levels of education, and tenure of residence. The emergency room users had lower socio-economic statuses, were five times as more likely to have the head of the family unemployed, and were likely to be from families with a total income of less than $5,000.

Thirty-seven percent (37%) of the ER population reported usually going to a physician when they needed care. Seventy percent (70%) came to the emergency service without first applying for other kinds of help. Most came on their own with no referral (55%). Six percent (6%) of the cases were classified as emergent, 36% as urgent and 56% as non-urgent. There were lower rates of non-urgent use among the youngest and oldest age groups, among whites compared to blacks, among those who had longer tenure in the city and for those with a private physician.

Weiss, G.L.

> 1972   "The influence of need and care and selected socio-demographic characteristics on the utilization of physician services." Unpub. M.S. thesis. Lafayette, Indiana: Department of Sociology, Purdue University.

This study introduces a kind of use-disability ratio, to monitor people's access to the use of needed medical services.

Data came from the 1971 CHAS-NORC national survey of health services utilization.

The use-disability ratio introduced here was computed by summing the total physician visits and total disability days experienced by a population in a two-week period, dividing the total visits by the total disability days and multiplying by 100. Appropriate, under-, and over-utilizers were also determined.

The indices were analyzed for the following variables: age, sex, marital status, family size, occupation, education, race, religion, income, insurance coverage, residence, region and distance.

Cross-tabulation of rates were used to report the findings.

The number of contacts per 100 disability days showed the importance of having health insurance coverage, a high income, good education, white skin and a white collar job, as each of these groups used more services relative to their need than their counterparts. The patterns described for under- over- and appropriate utilizers further confirmed these findings.

Welch, S., et al.

> 1973   "Some social and attitudinal correlates of health care among Mexican-Americans." *J. Health Soc. Behav.* 14 (September): 205-213.

This study was intended to ascertain the attitudes and health behaviors of a Mexican-American population in the state of Nebraska.

Data were collected from household interviews of a sample of Mexican-Americans drawn from four communities in two of the four counties that are centers of the Mexican-American population of Nebraska.

Some indicators of the utilization of medical care reported are the percent who had a family doctor, had seen a doctor within the last three months, had experienced times within the past year when they should have seen a doctor but did not, percent who had never seen a doctor, had had a polio vaccination, a tetanus shot, whose child had had a tetanus shot, had ever seen a dentist, whose child had ever seen a dentist, had seen a dentist within the last year, whose child had seen a dentist within the last year, had ever had his vision checked, and whose child had had his vision checked.

Respondent's attitudes toward doctors and medical care were reported, as was the method of financing their medical care, indicators of "closeness to Mexican society" (e.g., taking the interview in Spanish, number of years the respondent resided in the U.S., whether the respondent's parents were born in U.S., and the size of the Mexican-American community). Socio-economic indicators, such as the respondent's age, sex, education, income and number of years of residence in the community were also reported.

Cross-tabulation of percents and Pearson correlation coefficients were used to analyze the data.

It was hypothesized that socio-economic characteristics of the respondents would explain folk beliefs about doctors and medical care. Beliefs, however, were found to be most strongly related to the size of the Mexican-American community and not highly correlated with individuals' socio-economic attributes. Utilization of medical services was found to be related more to class and age than either to attitudes toward modern medicine or his closeness to "Mexican culture," however.

Wolfe, S. and R.F. Badgley

1972   "The family doctor." *Milb. Mem. Fund Quart.* 50 (April): 1-203.

The purpose of this study is to describe the role of the family doctor in improving accessibility and continuity of care.

Data were collected from clinic records of a Saskatoon medical group (the Saskatoon Community Health Services Association) in Saskatchewan, Canada.

A variety of utilization indices were reported — number of visits, number of doctors seen, usual family doctor, type of practitioner seen, etc.

Characteristics of the Saskatoon Plan and the membership itself were described.

AID, cross-tabulations, etc. were used to analyze the data.

The authors provide a comprehensive profile of the role of the family doctor, the advantages that accrue to him and to the patient of membership in a group practice setting and the policy implications that such a form of organization might have for the physicians and the consumer who wants comprehensive, continuous access to the medical care system.

Zola, I.K.

1966   "Culture and symptoms — an analysis of patients' presenting complaints." *ASR* 31 (October): 615-630.

The purpose of this study was to demonstrate that different ethnic groups may perceive and respond to symptoms differently.

The data were based on a comparison between 63 Italians (34 female, 25 male) and 81 Irish (42 female, 39 male), who were new admissions to the Eye, Ear, Nose and Throat and the Medical Clinics of Massachusetts General Hospital and the Massachusetts Eye and Ear Infirmary, seen between July, 1960, and February, 1961.

The nature, location, diffuseness, etc. of the presenting complaint was compared for the Irish and Italian patients.

A Chi-square test of significance was performed on the data.

The author concluded that "culture" — ethnic group membership — did affect the nature of complaints the patient presented to the physician. The Italians more often described pain with their complaint and said that their problem was of a diffuse, general nature. The Irish less often reported pain and described it as being rather specifically located. The author argues that the different illness behavior of Irish and Italians found in this sample may be the results of the different "defense mechanisms" prescribed by the culture of each — with the Irish handling their problems by denial and the Italians by dramatization.

6
Data Source Evaluation

Introduction

Data sources that provide information on our access concept on both a continuing and ad hoc basis are summarized.

The periodic data collection efforts reported include those of the American Hospital Association (AHA), American Medical Association (AMA), Center for Health Administration Studies (CHAS), the National Center for Health Statistics (NCHS) and the Social Security Administration (SSA). Surveys conducted by the Experimental Health Services Delivery Systems (EHSDS), the Office of Economic Opportunity (OEO) and the World Health Organization/International Collaborative Study of Medical Care Utilization (WHO/ICS-MCU) are also reported.

Information describing the data source (times of collection, population and/or sample, method of data collection); its relevance for the study of access (in terms of our framework); selected references; and the persons to be contacted for more information on each service are summarized.

The data source evaluations are arranged in alphabetical order by sponsoring agency.

American Hospital Association (AHA) Annual Survey of Hospitals

DESCRIPTION OF DATA SOURCE:

Times of collection (when and/or how often):

The Annual Survey of Hospitals has been conducted each year since 1946.

Population and/or sample:

Data are collected from AHA-registered hospitals and nonregistered hospitals. The former group includes about 7,200 hospitals in the United States and associated areas.

Method of data collection:

Questionnaires are sent to each of the hospitals from which information is sought. The National Center for Health Statistics distributes the questionnaires to nonregistered hospitals.

RELEVANCE FOR THE STUDY OF ACCESS:

The American Hospital Association is involved with collecting and processing data from a variety of periodic and ad hoc surveys of hospital facilities and utilization. The Annual Survey of Hospitals, however, provides continuing information on hospital facilities, use, financing and personnel, nationally, over time. In addition, the AHA is in the process of launching a study to compile existing data and collect new information, when necessary, on ambulatory (outpatient and emergency room) care available through hospitals.

I.   PROCESS INDICES

    A. *Characteristics of Health Delivery System*

       1. Resources
          a. Facilities — types of service available
          b. Number of beds (or bassinets) by type of service
          c. Changes in number of beds
          d. Financial data — revenue, expenses, assets
          e. Personnel on payroll
       2. Organization
          a. Approvals — accreditations, professional association approvals, etc.
          b. Classification — by control (government, etc.), services provided, average length of stay

    B. *Characteristics of Population-at-Risk*

Information in the Annual Survey is collected on the hospital, rather than individuals, as the elemental unit of analysis.

II. OUTCOME INDICES
A. *Utilization of Health Services*
1. Type
   a. Hospital
   b. Nursing and personal care homes
   c. Emergency care
   d. Other
2. Site — inpatient, outpatient, emergency room
3. Purpose
   a. Illness-related
      1) Curative — short-term hospitals
      2) Stabilizing — long-term hospitals
   b. Custodial
4. Time interval
   a. Contact — admissions
   b. Volume — average daily census, adjusted patient days (incorporates outpatient department visits), occupancy, length of stay, number of annual visits for various ambulatory care services, births, surgical operations
   c. Continuity — number of "referred" outpatient visits

SELECTED REFERENCES:

American Hospital Association
1973a *Hospital Statistics, 1972.* Chicago: American Hospital Association.
1973b *The 1973 AHA Guide to the Health Care Field.* Chicago: American Hospital Association. (Also see previous years of *Hospital Guide Issue.*)
1973c "Scheduled projects report, March, 1973." Chicago: Bureau of Research Services, American Hospital Association.

PERSONS TO BE CONTACTED ABOUT DATA SOURCE:

Bernard Ferber, Sc.D., Director
Bureau of Research Services
American Hospital Association
840 North Lake Shore Drive
Chicago, Illinois 60611

Alma Kuby, Director
Division of Data Collection
Bureau of Research Services
American Hospital Association
840 North Lake Shore Drive
Chicago, Illinois 60611

P. Joseph Phillip, Ph.D., Director
Division of Research
Bureau of Research Services
American Hospital Association
840 North Lake Shore Drive
Chicago, Illinois 60611

American Medical Association (AMA) Physician Masterfile

DESCRIPTION OF DATA SOURCE:

Times of collection (when and/or how often):

The Masterfile includes information on every known physician in the United States. A file is started on each individual upon entry into medical school or, in the case of foreign graduates, upon entry to the United States. The information in the file has been updated through periodic censuses of physicians. A complete census of all physicians is planned for every three years. In the interim years, the file will be kept current through a weekly updating system.

Population and/or sample:

The entire *known* physician population in the United States is the focus of the AMA Masterfile censuses.

Methods of data collection:

Record of Physicians' Professional Activities (PPA) questionnaires are used to collect information through the periodic censuses. Any indication from physicians, hospitals, government agencies, medical schools, state or county societies, specialty boards or societies of changes in physicians' professional address and/or status may signal the mailing of a PPA questionnaire for continual update of the Masterfile.

RELEVANCE FOR THE STUDY OF ACCESS:

This file provides information on a variety of characteristics of all practicing physicians in the United States. It is an excellent source of descriptive data on the physician manpower resource in the United States. Following is a summary of the basic variables available on the Masterfile.

I. PROCESS INDICES

   A. *Characteristics of Health Delivery System*
     1. Medical education number
       a. State or county of medical education
       b. Medical school of graduation
       c. Year of graduation
     2. Name of physician
     3. Sex
     4. Current professional mailing address
     5. Geographic codes
       a. State
       b. County
       c. City
       d. Zip code
     6. Birth date
     7. Birth place
     8. Citizenship and visa codes
     9. State licensure data
    10. National boards
    11. Major professional activity — type of practice
       a. Patient care
         1) Office based practice
         2) Hospital based practice
           a) Interns
           b) Residents
           c) Full-time physician staff
       b. Other professional activity
         1) Medical teaching
         2) Administration
         3) Research
         4) Other
       c. Inactive
       d. Not classified
    12. Specialty
       a. Primary
       b. Secondary
       c. Tertiary

13. Present employment
    a. Solo practice
    b. Partnership
    c. Arrangement
    d. Group practice
    e. Medical school
    f. Non-governmental hospital
    g. City or county government — hospital
    h. City or county government — other than hospital
    i. State government — hospital
    j. State government — other than hospital
    k. U.S. government — hospital
    l. U.S. government — other than hospital
    m. Other organizations
    n. Address unknown
    o. No classification
14. American specialty boards
15. Specialty societies
16. Current and former medical training
    a. Internship
    b. Residency
17. Current and former government service
18. Professional appointments
19. AMA membership

SELECTED REFERENCES:

American Medical Association

1973 *Data Base of the AMA Center for Health Services Research and Development.* Chicago: Center for Health Services Research and Development, American Medical Association.

1963- *Distribution of Physicians . . . in the United States.*
1971 Chicago: Center for Health Services Research and Development, American Medical Association.

PERSON TO BE CONTACTED ABOUT DATA SOURCE:

Chris N. Theodore, Director
Center for Health Services Research and Development
American Medical Association
535 North Dearborn Street
Chicago, Illinois 60610

American Medical Association (AMA) Periodic Survey of Physicians

DESCRIPTION OF DATA SOURCE:

Times of collection (when and/or how often):
The first Periodic Survey of Physicians (PSP) was conducted in 1966. Seven surveys have been completed (on an annual basis) and the eighth (1973) is currently in the field.

Population and/or sample:
The sample was selected from the AMA Masterfile. Each sample was randomly selected using a set of computer generated random numbers. The sizes of the samples were 3,544 physicians for PSP I; 5,265 for PSP II; 5,885 for PSP III; 5,052 for PSP IV; 7,563 for PSP V; 7,842 for PSP VI; and 9,160 for PSP VII. PSP VIII differs somewhat from previous PSP's in that it includes three separate samples — the main sample of 7,500 physicians and samples of 1,000 each of women physicians and foreign medical graduates.

Methods of data collection:
PSP questionnaires are mailed to each of the physicians sampled. A series of follow-up requests are sent to nonrespondents at three week intervals. In the 1973 PSP, all women physicians surveyed received a supplementary sheet soliciting special information on factors which may have influenced the nature of their practice.

RELEVANCE FOR THE STUDY OF ACCESS:

This file provides information on the practice and patient characteristics of a random sample of physicians in the United States. Though information is collected on patients and utilization rates, the physician's practice, rather than the individual himself, is the elemental unit of analysis.

I.   PROCESS INDICES

    A. *Characteristics of Health Delivery System*
        1. Practice characteristics
            a. Primary specialty
            b. Number of years in practice
            c. Number of years in specialty
            d. Number of years in training
            e. Type of practice (solo, group, etc.)
            f. Source of professional income (fee-for-service, etc.)

     g. Number of rooms which comprise the working environment
     h. Hospital staff privileges (number and type)
     i. Ownership of hospital or nursing home
  2. Hours, weeks worked
     a. Number of weeks practiced per year
     b. Number of hours practiced per week
     c. Number of hours in patient care per week
     d. Number of hours "on call"
     e. Number of hours per week devoted to personnel management and administration
     f. Number of hours per week spent in operating, delivery, and labor rooms
  3. Professional income
     a. Gross income from medical practice
     b. Collection ratio
     c. Percent of gross income from uninsured, insured at fee-for-service capitation
     d. Percent of gross income from lab, x-ray services
     e. Percent of gross income from solo, salary, share of fee-for-service
  4. Professional expenses (tax deductible)
     a. Total professional expenses
     b. Salaries and wages
       1) Physicians
       2) Non-physicians
     c. Plant and facilities
       1) Rent or mortgage
       2) Fuel and utilities
       3) Insurance
       4) Real estate taxes
     d. Professional liability insurance
     e. Outside lab and x-ray
     f. Drugs and medical supplies
     g. Legal, accounting and management
     h. Current value of medical assets
     i. Average age of office, medical equipment
  5. Professional fees
     a. Data collected on fees for 18 procedures (PSP #II, IV, V, VI)
     b. Data collected on fees for 12 procedures (PSP #VII)

    6. Ancillary personnel
      a. Number of hours worked per week
      b. Number of weeks worked per year
      c. Number of full-time equivalents (FTE) employed
      d. Salary paid per FTE
      e. Percent of time ten selected tasks performed by allied health personnel
      f. Type of allied health personnel likely to perform ten selected tasks

B. *Characteristics of Population-at-Risk*
    1. Predisposing
      a. Immutable
        1) Age
        2) Sex

    2. Enabling
      a. Mutable
        1) Income
        2) Medicaid eligibility
        3) Referrals

II. OUTCOME INDICES

A. *Utilization*
    1. Number of patient visits per week (office, hospital, nursing home, other)
    2. Number of times 12 selected procedures are performed per week
    3. Number of times an average patient is seen in year

SELECTED REFERENCES:

American Medical Association

1973 *Data Base of the AMA Center for Health Services Research and Development.* Chicago: Center for Health Services Research and Development, American Medical Association.

1971- *Reference Data on the Profile of Medical Practice.*
1973 Chicago: Center for Health Services Research and Development, American Medical Association.

PERSON TO BE CONTACTED ABOUT DATA SOURCE:

Chris N. Theodore, Director
Center for Health Services Research and Development
American Medical Association
535 North Dearborn Street
Chicago, Illinois 60610

American Medical Association (AMA) Group Practice File

DESCRIPTION OF DATA SOURCE:

Times of collection (when and/or how often):

In 1965 the AMA conducted "The Register of Group Practice" survey. In 1969 a census of all known groups was conducted. In 1971 as a part of a collaborative study of the AMA and the University of Southern California, a survey of 2,000 medical groups was undertaken. The data from these three sources were used to construct the AMA Group Practice File.

Population and/or sample:

Using the group practice surveys and the AMA Physician Masterfile, two basic subfiles are in the process of being created within the AMA Group Practice File — characteristics of 1) group practices, and 2) group practice physicians.

Methods of data collection:

The AMA Physician Masterfile provides data on all group practice physicians. Supplementary survey work is being planned to provide data on all known group practices.

RELEVANCE FOR THE STUDY OF ACCESS:

This file provides information on a variety of characteristics of group practices and group practice physicians. Though information is provided on utilization rates, the physician and his practice, rather than the individual himself, is the elemental unit of analysis.

I.   PROCESS INDICES

A. *Characteristics of Health Delivery System*
    1. Practice characteristics
        a. Name and address of group
        b. Date and size at formation of group
        c. Fields of practice

d. Number of and kinds of physicians and other personnel
e. Form of organization — single ownership, partnership, corporation, etc.
f. Ownership of office space
g. Organization of record keeping
h. Size of community in which practice is located
i. Affiliations with other organizations (hospitals, etc.)
j. Type of service provided
k. Type of administrator and nature of board
l. Method of payment for services rendered
m. Number of prepaid subscribers
n. Rooms and amount of space that comprise working environment

2. Hours, weeks worked
a. Weeks worked by respective personnel
b. Hours per week worked by respective personnel

3. Entry
a. Appointment waiting time for typical patient
b. Office waiting time for typical patient

4. Professional income
a. Total receipts from medical practice
b. Collection ratio
c. Percent of gross income from uninsured, insured or fee-for-service capitation
d. Percent of gross income from lab, x-ray services
e. Percent of gross income from prepayment

5. Professional expenses (tax deductible)
a. Total professional expenses
b. Salaries and wages
   a) Physicians
   2) Non-physicians
c. Plants and facilities
d. Professional liability insurance
e. Outside lab and x-ray
f. Drugs and medical supplies
g. Legal, accounting and management
h. Current value of group's medical assets
i. Average age of practice-related assets

6. Professional fees
a. Data collected on fees for 12 procedures

7. Ancillary personnel
   a. Number of hours worked per week
   b. Number of weeks worked per year
   c. Number of full-time equivalents (FTE) employed
   d. Salary paid per FTE

II.   OUTCOME INDICES

   A. *Utilization*
      1. Number of patient visits per week (office, hospital, nursing home, other)
      2. Percent of visits reported above that were to medical, surgical or other specialist, or to a non-physician
      3. Number of times an average patient is seen in year
      4. Average number of visits per prepaid subscriber in year

SELECTED REFERENCES:

American Medical Association
   1973 *Data Base of the AMA Center for Health Services Research and Development.* Chicago: Center for Health Services Research and Development, American Medical Association.

   1965, *(Survey of) Medical Groups in the United States.* Chicago:
   1969   Center for Health Services Research and Development, American Medical Association.

PERSON TO BE CONTACTED ABOUT DATA SOURCE:

Chris N. Theodore, Director
Center for Health Services Research and Development
American Medical Association
535 North Dearborn Street
Chicago, Illinois 60610

Center for Health Administration Studies (Health Information Foundation) - National Opinion Research Center — CHAS (HIF) - NORC — nationwide surveys of health services utilization and expenditures

DESCRIPTION OF DATA SOURCE:

Times of collection (when and/or how often):
There have been four (4) CHAS (HIF) - NORC nationwide surveys of health services utilization and expenditures, conducted in July, 1953; May, 1958; January-March, 1964; and January-March, 1971.

Population and/or sample:

1953 survey. An area probability sample was used in this survey. It was drawn by the same methods as those used by the Bureau of the Census in the Current Population Survey. There were 2,809 families that comprised 8,846 individuals, representing a national sample of the United States.

1958 study. The sample design for this survey was, in essence, identical to that of the 1953 survey through the segment-selection stage. A screening procedure was employed to over-sample families with high medical expenditures. It yielded information on 9,546 members of 2,941 families.

1964 study. Attempts were made to insure that the methodology employed was comparable to the 1953 and 1958 studies. Data were collected from 2,367 families for 7,803 individuals.

1971 study. The master sample was essentially the same as that used in the 1964 study. It was not a self-weighting area probability sample of U.S. population, however. It over-represented people of special concern in health policy formulation, including those with low incomes, living in central cities, the rural population, and persons 66 and over. A complex weighting scheme was employed to make the sample more closely representative of the United States population. There were 3,880 families consisting of 11,619 individuals in the sample. The weighted sample size was 56,815 persons.

Methods of data collection:

In each of the studies, household interview of family members and verification forms sent to hospitals, were the methods used to collect data. In 1964, a verification of all insurance coverage was attempted through insurance and employers. More limited verifications of coverage had been carried out in 1953 and 1958. In 1971, verifications of insurance claims and physician care were carried out in addition to the verifications done in the earlier studies.

RELEVANCE FOR THE STUDY OF ACCESS:

Collection of information on national samples of the population, with respect to their utilization and expenditures for health care, permits comparisons over time of the population's access to the health care system.

I.   PROCESS INDICES

   A. *Characteristics of Health Delivery System*

     Questions included in the survey, that reflect characteristics of the health delivery system, are actually asked of individuals. They appear as "enabling" characteristics of the population-at-risk.

     Information on the resources and organization of the delivery system itself as the unit of analysis — physician-population ratios (1964, 1971), board certification of physicians (1964, 1971), average monthly number of Medicaid recipients in a state (1971), etc., are included in the analysis of these data. This information, however, was obtained from other sources (AMA, SSA, etc.).

   B. *Characteristics of Population-at-Risk*

     1. Predisposing

       a. Mutable

         1) General health care beliefs and attitudes (1964, 1971)

         2) Knowledge and sources of health care information (1964, 1971)

       b. Immutable

         1) Age (1953, 1958, 1964, 1971)

         2) Sex (1953, 1958, 1964, 1971)

         3) Marital status (1953, 1958, 1964, 1971)

         4) Previous health behavior (1953, 1958, 1964, 1971)

         5) Education (1953, 1958, 1964, 1971)

         6) Race or ethnicity (1953, 1958, 1964, 1971)

         7) Family size and composition (1953, 1958, 1964, 1971)

         8) Religion (1953, 1958, 1964, 1971)

         9) Residential mobility (1953, 1958, 1964, 1971)

     2. Enabling

       a. Mutable

         1) Socioeconomic status and occupation (1953, 1958, 1964, 1971)

         2) Income and sources of income (1953, 1958, 1964, 1971)

         3) Insurance coverage — type of payer, extent of coverage, method of payment (1953, 1958, 1964, 1971)

   4) Price of medical services (1953, 1958, 1964, 1971)
   5) Organization of services — solo or group practice
      (1971)
   6) Regular source of care (1964, 1971)
   7) Ease of getting to regular source of care — method
      of transportation, travel time, appointment or
      walk-in visit, appointment waiting time, office wait-
      ing time (1971)
   8) Availability of health resources — physician-
      population, hospital-population ratios, etc. (1964,
      1971); level of Medicaid benefits available per state
      (1971)
3. Need
   a. Perceived
      1) Health status — general evaluation (1964, 1971);
         worry, pain (1971)
      2) Symptoms of illness (1964, 1971)
      3) Disability days — bed days, restricted activity days
         in two weeks (1971) and year (1964, 1971)
   b. Evaluated
      1) Medically-defined need — symptom and diagnoses
         severity ratings (1971)
      2) Diagnosis — conditions (1953, 1958, 1964, 1971)
      3) Surgery (1953, 1958, 1964, 1971)

II.   OUTCOME INDICES

A. *Utilization of Health Services*
   1. Type
      a. Hospital (1953, 1958, 1964, 1971)
      b. Physician — general practitioner, specialist, chirop-
         ractor, chiropodist-podiatrist, optometrist (1953, 1958,
         1964, 1971)
      c. Dentist (1953, 1958, 1964, 1971)
      d. Nursing and personal care homes (1953, 1958, 1964,
         1971)
      e. Prescribed and nonprescribed drugs — druggist (1953,
         1958, 1964, 1971)
      f. Appliances — vision aids (1953, 1958, 1964, 1971)
      g. Home care (1953, 1958, 1964, 1971)
      h. Emergency care (1953, 1958, 1964, 1971)

      i. Other — x-rays, lab tests, physical therapist, clinical psychologist, visiting nurse, naturopath-naprapath, homeopath, Christian Science practitioner, physician's assistant, nurse (1953, 1958, 1964, 1971)

  2. Site — home; office or private clinic; hospital inpatient, outpatient, emergency room; industrial, school, camp, or college health service, other clinic or neighborhood health center (1953, 1958, 1964, 1971)

  3. Purpose

    a. Preventive

      1) General exam — time interval and reason (1964, 1971)

      2) Obstetrical — number and trimester of visits for pregnancy (1953, 1958, 1964, 1971)

      3) Immunizations — polio vaccine, flu shots, TB x-ray (1964, 1971)

    b. Illness-related

      1) Curative — minor illnesses (1953, 1958, 1964, 1971)

      2) Stabilizing — major illnesses (1953, 1958, 1964, 1971)

    c. Custodial (1953, 1958, 1964, 1971)

  4. Time interval

    a. Contact — did or did not see a doctor in two weeks (year); did or did not see dentist in year; was or was not admitted to hospital in past year, etc. (1953, 1958, 1964, 1971)

    b. Volume — number of doctor, dentist visits; number of hospital admissions and length of stay; expenditures; etc. (1953, 1958, 1964, 1971)

    c. Continuity — *episodes* of illness — provider who rendered most care (1971); number of providers and visits per episode (1953, 1958, 1964, 1971); reason for patient going to respective providers (1971)

B. *Consumer Satisfaction*

Level of satisfaction (in general) with overall quality of care, waiting time, availability on weekends, ease of getting to care, out-of-pocket costs for care, information given about what was wrong, . . . about what you should do at home to treat illness, courtesy and consideration shown by doctors, . . . by nurses, follow-up care, concern of doctors for overall health, getting all of needs taken care of at one place, information available for choosing physician (1971).

SELECTED REFERENCES:

Andersen, R.

1968   *A Behavioral Model of Families' Use of Health Services.* Research Series No. 25. Chicago: Center for Health Administration Studies, University of Chicago.

Andersen, R. and O. W. Anderson

1967   *A Decade of Health Services.* Chicago: University of Chicago Press.

Andersen, R. and J. Kravits

1971   "Disability days and physician contact for the two week period preceding the interview date by age, sex, race, residence, and family income." Preliminary Report No. 1 of research conducted under contract No. HSM 110-70-392, NCHSRD. Chicago: Center for Health Administration Studies, University of Chicago.

Andersen, R. and J. Newman

1973   "Societal and individual determinants of medical care utilization." *Milb. Mem. Fund Quart.* 51 (Winter): 95-124.

Andersen, R., et al.

1972   *Health Service Use: National Trends and Variations — 1953-1971.* Washington: National Center for Health Services Research and Development, U.S. Dept. HEW Publication No. (HSM) 73-3004.

1973   *Expenditures for Personal Health Services: National Trends and Variations — 1953-1970.* Washington: Bureau of Health Services Research and Evaluation, U.S. Dept. HEW Publication No. (HRA) 74-3105.

1971   "The public's view of the crisis in medical care: an impetus for changing delivery systems?" *Econ. & Bus. Bulletin* 24, (Fall): 44-52.

Anderson, O. W.

1963   "The utilization of health services." In Freeman, H. E., et al. (eds.) *Handbook of Medical Sociology.* Englewood Cliffs, New Jersey: Prentice-Hall.

Anderson, O. W. and R. Andersen

1972   "Patterns of use of health services." In Freeman, H. E. et al. (eds.) *Handbook of Medical Sociology.* Englewood Cliffs, New Jersey: Prentice-Hall.

Anderson, O. W. and J. J. Feldman

1956   *Family Medical Costs and Voluntary Health Insurance: A Nationwide Survey.* New York: McGraw Hill Book Co., Inc.

Anderson, O. W., et al.

1963   *Changes in Family Medical Care Expenditures and Voluntary Health Insurance.* Cambridge: Harvard University Press.

1960   *Family Expenditure Patterns for Personal Health Services — 1953 and 1958: Nationwide Surveys,* Research Series No. 14. Chicago: Center for Health Administration Studies, University of Chicago.

PERSONS TO BE CONTACTED ABOUT DATA SOURCE:

Odin W. Anderson, Ph.D.
Professor and Director
Center for Health Administration Studies
University of Chicago
5720 South Woodlawn Avenue
Chicago, Illinois 60637

Ronald Andersen, Ph.D.
Research Associate and Associate Professor
Center for Health Administration Studies
University of Chicago
5720 South Woodlawn Avenue
Chicago, Illinois 60637

Experimental Health Services Delivery Systems (EHSDS) household surveys, funded by the National Center for Health Services Research and Development (NCHSRD)

DESCRIPTION OF DATA SOURCE:

Times of collection (when and/or how often):
Baseline surveys were conducted in the different EHSDS communities from summer, 1972, through spring, 1973.

Population and/or sample:
The eighteen EHSDS communities in which the surveys were conducted were Alabama, Arkansas, Avoca, Boise, Delaware, East Los Angeles, Jacksonville, Kentucky, Lubbock, Memphis, Mon Valley, New Haven, New York-Pennsylvania, Philadelphia, Rapid City, St. Louis, Tucson and Vermont. The sampling design in each community varied, depending upon local needs and requirements. Purdue University's Health Services Research and Training Program serves as the archive for these data and has compiled detailed documentation of the sampling design, etc., in each community.

Method of data collection:
Both household and telephone interviews were used to collect the data. Some communities did assemble information on the characteristics of the delivery systems in the respective areas. Communities were also asked to put ambulatory care and hospital discharge data components into place, but few have done so.

RELEVANCE FOR THE STUDY OF ACCESS:

This series of surveys were taken in communities in which innovations in the organization and delivery of medical care were to be introduced. These surveys were to collect baseline information on the population-at-risk's access to medical care, especially their need for and use of services, that could be incorporated into an "index of access" to care, the use-need discrepancy ratio. The EHSDS experience is a useful model for understanding how the impact of different programs on a community's access to care might be evaluated.

I.   PROCESS INDICES

     A. *Characteristics of Health Delivery System*
        Some communities did collect information on the resources and organization of the delivery system in the area. There were no systematic guidelines for collecting these data, however.

     B. *Characteristics of Population-at-Risk*
        1. Predisposing
           a. Mutable
              1) General health care beliefs and attitudes (optional)
           b. Immutable
              1) Age
              2) Sex
              3) Marital status
              4) Education
              5) Race or ethnicity
              6) Family size and composition

        2. Enabling
           a. Mutable
              1) Socioeconomic status and occupation
              2) Income
              3) Insurance coverage — type of payer, extent of coverage
              4) Price of medical services (optional)
              5) Regular source of care
              6) Ease of getting to regular source of care — travel time (plus, series of optional questions on office waiting time, whether doctor makes house calls, etc.)
           b. Immutable
              1) Region — study area
              2) Residence

        3. Need
           a. Perceived
              1) Disability days — bed days in two weeks and year, restricted activity days in two weeks and condition causing disability days in two weeks
              2) Chronic activity limitation — presence of chronic condition and whether there is limitation of activity.

II. OUTCOME INDICES

A. *Utilization of Health Services*
   1. Type
      a. Hospital
      b. Physician
      c. Dentist (optional)
   2. Site — office; hospital inpatient, outpatient, emergency room, industrial clinic; other clinic; telephone
   3. Purpose
      a. Illness-related
         1) Curative — acute disability
         2) Stabilizing — chronic disability
   4. Time interval
      a. Contact — did or did not see a doctor in two weeks (or year); did or did not see dentist in past year (optional); was or was not admitted to hospital in past year
      b. Volume — number of doctor, dentist (optional) visits; number of hospital admissions and length of stay

B. *Consumer Satisfaction*

   Level of satisfaction (in general) from items in 1971 CHAS survey; optional questions on perceived barriers to access regarding travel times, costs, waiting times, physician's concern, etc., from NCHS, WHO/ICS-MCU, CHAS surveys; reasons cited for not seeing a doctor when respondent felt he *should* (all these satisfaction items were optional).

SELECTED REFERENCES:

Health Services Research and Training Program
   1972 *Health Services Data System: The Family Health Survey.* Lafayette, Indiana: Health Services Research and Training Program, Purdue University.

U.S. Department of Health, Education, and Welfare
   1971 *Experimental Health Services Delivery Systems.* Washington: National Center for Health Services Research and Development.

PERSON TO BE CONTACTED ABOUT DATA SOURCE:

Robert Eichhorn, Ph.D., Director
Health Services Research and Training Program
303 Russell St.
Lafayette, Indiana 47906

National Center for Health Statistics-Health Interview Survey (NCHS-HIS)

DESCRIPTION OF DATA SOURCE:

Times of collection (when and/or how often):

Household interviews are conducted on a continuing basis each week on a probability sample of the nation's population. The Health Interview Survey has been conducted every year since 1957.

Population and/or sample:

Samples for successive weeks of the survey can be combined into larger samples to obtain data for a quarter, a year, or a larger period of time. Data collected over a year can be presented as annual estimates which are free of seasonal biases.

The interview sample is a highly stratified, multi-stage probability design. The first stage consists of an area sample drawn from about 1,900 geographically defined primary sampling units (PSU's) into which the nation has been divided. Second and subsequent stages consist of a series of steps for further subsampling within the chosen PSU's. Some 42,000 households provide data on about 134,000 persons in this survey.

Methods of data collection:

Household interviews of the sample population constitutes the means of collecting information.

RELEVANCE FOR THE STUDY OF ACCESS:

This survey provides valuable baseline information, over time, for the utilization of and need for care for the population nationally.[1]

I.   PROCESS INDICES

A. *Characteristics of Health Delivery System*

The Health Interview Survey primarily provides information on the characteristics and utilization experience of the population-at-risk. The characteristics of the delivery system about which information are sought are included as "enabling" characteristics of the population.

---

[1]Though a variety of detailed information on individuals' health care seeking are collected in the Health Interview Survey, only the general categories relevant to our access concept (and the years in which information on them were collected) will be cited.

B. *Characteristics of Population-at-Risk*
   1. Predisposing
      a. Immutable
         1) Age (1958-1973)
         2) Sex (1958-1973)
         3) Marital status (1958-1973)
         4) Previous health behavior (1958-1973)
         5) Education (1958-1973)
         6) Race or ethnicity (1958-1973)
         7) Family size and composition (1958-1973)
   2. Enabling
      a. Mutable
         1) Socioeconomic status (1960-1973) and occupation (1962, 1963, 1966-1973)
         2) Income and source of income (1958-1973)
         3) Insurance coverage — type of payer, extent of coverage, method of payment (1960, 1963, 1968, 1970, 1972)
         4) Price of medical services (1960, 1963, 1968, 1970, 1972)
         5) Organization of services — solo or group practice (1970, 1972)
         6) Regular source of care (1973)
         7) Ease of getting to care — travel time (1969, 1973); office waiting time (1969, 1973); appointment or not and problems with making it (1969, 1973); reasons cited for problems in getting medical care — doctor availability, money, didn't know where to go (1973)
      b. Immutable
         1) Region (1958-1973)
         2) Residence (1958-1973)
   3. Need
      a. Perceived
         1) Disability days — restricted activity, bed, work-loss and school-loss days in two weeks and bed days in past year and condition causing disability (1958-1973)
         2) Chronic activity limitation (1958-1973)
      b. Evaluated
         1) Diagnosis — conditions (general), accidents and injuries (1958-1973); edentulousness (1958, 1971);

diabetes (1965); visual impairments (1964-1967, 1971-1973); hearing impairments (1963, 1971); arthritis (1969); smoking (1965, 1966, 1970)
   2) Surgery (1958-1973)

II.   OUTCOME INDICES

   A. *Utilization of Health Services*
     1. Type
       a. Hospital (1958-1973)
       b. Physician — type of specialist (1958-1973)
       c. Dentist (1958, 1964, 1969-1972)
       d. Nursing and personal care homes (1958-1973)
       e. Prescribed and nonprescribed drugs (1965, 1973)
       f. Appliances — visual aids (1966); other aids (1959, 1969)
       g. Home care (1959, 1967, 1968)
       h. Emergency care (1972, 1973)
       i. Other — x-rays (1961, 1964, 1970)
     2. Site — home; office or private clinic; hospital inpatient, outpatient, emergency room; company or industrial clinic; other; telephone (1958, 1959, 1964, 1966-1973)
     3. Purpose
       a. Preventive
         1) General exam — time interval and reason (1964, 1973)
         2) Obstetrical — number and trimester of visits for pregnancy and postnatal care (1973)
         3) Tests — EKG, eye pressure test for glaucoma, chest x-ray, Pap smear, breast examination (1973)
       b. Illness-related
         1) Curative — acute conditions (1958-1973)
         2) Stabilizing — chronic conditions (1958-1973)
       c. Custodial (1958-1973)
     4. Time interval
       a. Contact — did or did not see a physician in two weeks or year (for condition) (1958-1973); did not see dentist in two weeks or year (1958, 1959, 1964, 1969-1973); was or was not hospitalized in past two weeks or year (1958-1973); etc.
       b. Volume — number of doctor visits, number of dentist visits, number of hospital admissions and length of

stay, expenditures (1963, 1966, 1971), etc.
   c. Continuity — getting advice from source prior to consulting with physician, how doctor was chosen, doctor as regular source of care, return visit requested and compliance, medicine prescribed and compliance, referred to another doctor and compliance, delay and reasons for delay — couldn't get an appointment, didn't have money, etc. (1973)

B. *Consumer Satisfaction*
   Relative importance of aspects of medical care process — convenient office hours, doctor knowing name, doctor's explanation of what is wrong, doctor's charges, staff courtesy, time to get to office, getting an appointment when wanted, amount of time doctor spends with you, amount of time to pay bill; problems and degree of difficulty in making appointment, getting there, waiting time, reaching doctor by phone; general satisfaction with treatment or care received (1973)

SELECTED REFERENCES:

National Center for Health Statistics
   1963- Series 10. *Data from the Health Interview Survey*
   1974 (Numbers 1-91). Washington: National Center for Health Statistics.

PERSON TO BE CONTACTED ABOUT DATA SOURCE:

Elijah L. White, Director
Division of Health Interview Statistics
National Center for Health Statistics
Parklawn Building
5600 Fishers Lane
Rockville, Maryland 20852

National Center for Health Statistics Health Records Survey, which includes 1) Master Facility Inventory (MFI), 2) Complement Survey, 3) Hospital Discharge Survey (HDS), 4) Institutional Population Survey, and 5) special ad hoc surveys

DESCRIPTION OF DATA SOURCE:

1) The Master Facility Inventory is a comprehensive file of those facilities in the United States which provide medical, nursing, per-

sonal or custodial care to groups of unrelated persons on an inpatient basis. In order to keep the MFI current, the entire list of inpatient health facilities is surveyed biennially by mail.

2) The Complement Survey is used to locate facilities that are not currently included in the Master Facility Inventory. The Health Interview Survey (HIS) is routinely conducted across the nation. During the course of the HIS interviewer's regular assignments, a list is made of the names and addresses of all establishments in the blocks or segments of PSU's in which the interviews are conducted. Each establishment identified in the Complement Survey that is not on the Master Facility list is sent a MFI questionnaire, so it can be properly classified.

3) The Hospital Discharge Survey (HDS) is a continuing survey (since 1964) of short-stay hospitals to obtain statistics on the use of services, on the services provided in hospitals and the characteristics of patients. The survey involves a two-stage probability sample — the first being a sampling of short-term hospitals and the second-stage a sampling of discharges. Information from the discharges is copied on standard hospital discharge abstract forms.

4) The Institutional Population Survey is based on a stratified, multi-stage probability sample of resident institutions which provide psychiatric, medical, nursing, and personal care to the aged, infirm, or chronically ill. The survey is conducted by mail in establishments with less than 300 beds. For larger homes and hospitals, personal visits are made. The Master Facility Inventory of institutions provided the sampling frame for the survey.

5) The special ad hoc surveys collect information on the health of institutional residents, staffing patterns, etc.

RELEVANCE FOR THE STUDY OF ACCESS:

These data sources provide information on the characteristics and distribution of medical care resources in the United States. In reporting utilization rates in the Hospital Discharge and Institutional Population Surveys, the institutions, rather than the individuals themselves, are the primary sources of information (unlike the Health Interview Survey).

The Master Facility Inventory includes 1) a list of names and addresses of all hospitals in the United States with six or more beds, as well as all resident institutions, except for nursing or personal care homes with less than three beds, and 2) information which describes each with respect to their size, type and current status of business.

The Hospital Discharge Survey provides statistics on the utilization of short-stay hospitals in the United States, including information on the characteristics of the patients, on the conditions causing hospitalization, on operations performed, and on other services provided by the hospital.

The Institutional Population Surveys provide statistics on the health of residents in institutions and on factors relating to their care, including the training of staff, the provision of services, and the availability of facilities. Certain data complementary to the Health Interview Survey, about the noninstitutional population, such as their chronic conditions, impairments and the use of prosthetic devices have been collected, as has information on the types of nursing and personal services provided to patients and the experience and special training of the staff to provide care to the aged.

SELECTED REFERENCES:

National Center for Health Statistics

1965- Series 12. *Data from the Institutional Population Surveys*
1973   (Number 1-21). Washington: National Center for Health Statistics.

1966- Series 13. *Data from the Hospital Discharge Survey*
1974   (Numbers 1-14). Washington: National Center for Health Statistics.

1971 *Health Resource Statistics*. Washington: National Center for Health Statistics, U.S. Dept. HEW Publication No. (HSM) 72-1509.

PERSONS TO BE CONTACTED ABOUT DATA SOURCE:

Siegfried A. Hoermann, Director
Division of Health Resources Statistics
National Center for Health Statistics
Parklawn Building
5600 Fishers Lane
Rockville, Maryland 20852

G. Gloria Hollis, Chief
Health Facilities Statistics Branch
Division of Health Resources Statistics
National Center for Health Statistics
Parklawn Building
5600 Fishers Lane
Rockville, Maryland 20852

Grace K. White, Chief
Hospital Discharge Survey Branch
Division of Health Resources Statistics
National Center for Health Statistics
Parklawn Building
5600 Fishers Lane
Rockville, Maryland 20852

National Center for Health Statistics-Health Resources Data from 1) Medical Manpower Surveys, and 2) National Ambulatory Medical Care Survey (NAMCS)

DESCRIPTION OF DATA SOURCE:

1) The primary sources of health manpower data are professional organizations. Some of the data collection efforts are supported entirely by the professional organizations themselves, as with the American Medical Association, or they may be assisted by the NIH Bureau of Health Manpower Education, as are the American Dental Association and the American Nurses Association. NCHS has attempted to compile information from these sources and has, itself, recently conducted surveys of pharmacists, opticians and optometrists.

2) The National Ambulatory Medical Care Survey was launched in May, 1973. A sample of physicians are asked to complete a Patient Record for a systematic sample of approximately ten patients each day he practices, during a randomly assigned reporting week. By the end of the first year of the survey, about 1,700 physicians will have been asked to participate.

RELEVANCE FOR THE STUDY OF ACCESS:

These data provide information on the characteristics and distribution of health manpower resources and (in the case of the NAMCS) information on patient and provider characteristics and utilization, with the physician's practice itself as the elemental sampling unit.

The Medical Manpower Surveys conducted by NCHS and the data from the professional organizations (AMA, ANA, etc.) that NCHS has compiled, contain information on the geographic location, age, sex, education, type and place of employment, training, specialties, activities, time spent at work, etc., for the various kinds of medical care professionals.

The NAMCS obtains information on participating physicians' specialty, staff composition and whether his practice is a solo, partnership or group arrangement. The Patient Record Form collects data on the patient's age, sex, race, presenting symptoms or complaints, seriousness of the problem, whether patient was seen before, major reason(s) for the visit, physician's principal diagnosis, treatment provided, disposition of case and duration of the visit.

SELECTED REFERENCES:

DeLozier, J. E.

> 1974 "The design and methods of the National Ambulatory Medical Care Survey," *Medical Group Management* (January-February): 5-7.

National Center for Health Statistics

> 1968- Series 14. *Data on Health Resources: Manpower and*
> 1973 *Facilities* (Numbers 1-10). Washington: National Center for Health Statistics.

PERSONS TO BE CONTACTED ABOUT DATA SOURCE:

Siegfried A. Hoermann, Director
Division of Health Resources Statistics
National Center for Health Statistics
Parklawn Building
5600 Fishers Lane
Rockville, Maryland 20852

Harry S. Mount, Chief
Health Manpower Statistics Branch
Division of Health Resources Statistics
National Center for Health Statistics
Parklawn Building
5600 Fishers Lane
Rockville, Maryland 20852

James E. DeLozier, Statistician
Division of Health Resources Statistics
National Center for Health Statistics
Parklawn Building
5600 Fishers Lane
Rockville, Maryland 20852

National Center for Health Statistics Health (and Nutrition) Examination Survey (HANES)

DESCRIPTION OF DATA SOURCE:

The Health Examination Surveys are studies of the health of the population using direct physical examinations, clinical and laboratory tests, and other measurements. Three survey cycles have been completed. They have covered 1) the adult population (1959-1962), 2) children ages 6-11 (1963-1965), and 3) youths, ages 12-16 (1966-1970). The Health and Nutrition Examination Survey (HANES), the cycle now in progress, covers the population 1-74 years of age, and gives special emphasis to unmet health needs and nutritional status. Each cycle has used a probability sample. For the first three, the samples included 6,000 to 8,000 persons; in the current cycle, it is planned to examine some 30,000 individuals.

RELEVANCE FOR THE STUDY OF ACCESS:

This survey provides direct clinical information on the health status of the population and also relevant properties of the population-at-risk, and their utilization of and satisfaction with care.

Information collected on the individuals themselves include their attitudes about health care and physician visits, housing, education, occupation, ethnicity, income, insurance coverage, time to get an appointment, time to arrive at physician's office, and waiting time. Information on the individuals' perceptions of health and detailed clinical data are collected.

Information is collected on doctor and dentist visits and hospitalizations and when general exams and immunizations were last received.

Satisfaction with the last visit to the doctor, whether or not the waiting time was too long, etc., were also elicited.

SELECTED REFERENCES:

National Center for Health Statistics
    1964- Series 11. *Data from the Health Examination Survey.*
    1974 (Numbers 1-141). Washington: National Center for Health Statistics.

PERSON TO BE CONTACTED ABOUT DATA SOURCE:

Arthur J. McDowell, Director
Division of Health Examination Statistics
National Center for Health Statistics
Parklawn Building
5600 Fishers Lane
Rockville, Maryland 20852

Office of Economic Opportunity (OEO) neighborhood health center baseline surveys

DESCRIPTION OF DATA SOURCE:

Times of collection (when and/or how often):
The surveys were conducted in several communities in 1968-1969, prior to the introduction of neighborhood health centers in each area.

Population and/or sample:
Efforts were made to sample low-income target populations in each area. The National Opinion Research Center (NORC) drew the samples for the following communities: Roxbury, Bedford-Stuyvesant, Red Hook, Southeast Philadelphia, Cardoza, Charleston, Atlanta, Mission East Palo Alto, and Wisconsin (five counties). The University of Montana and Montana State College conducted the survey of the 16 Montana counties.

Method of data collection:
Household interviews were used to collect the information in each community.

RELEVANCE FOR THE STUDY OF ACCESS:

This survey was collected to provide baseline data on a low-income population's "access" to medical care prior to the introduction of neighborhood health centers in their communities. As such, it may be seen as part of a strategy to evaluate the impact of changes in the delivery system on a target population's access to the system.

I. PROCESS INDICES

A. *Characteristics of Health Delivery System*
Some information was collected on the existing resources, etc., in the different communities, but there were no systematic guidelines for the collection of these data.

Questions included in the survey, that reflect characteristics of the delivery system, appear as "enabling" characteristics of the population-at-risk.

B. *Characteristics of Population-at-Risk*
  1. Predisposing
    a. Immutable
      1) Age
      2) Sex
      3) Marital status
      4) Previous health behavior
      5) Education
      6) Race or ethnicity
      7) Family size and composition
      8) Residential mobility

  2. Enabling
    a. Mutable
      1) Socioeconomic status and occupation — usual activity
      2) Income and sources of income
      3) Insurance coverage — type of payer (special emphasis on Medicaid and Medicare), extent of coverage, method of payment
      4) Organization — solo or group practice
      5) Regular source of care
      6) Ease of getting to regular source of care — travel time (also asked for dentists), office waiting time
    b. Immutable
      1) Region — study area
      2) Residence

  3. Need
    a. Perceived
      1) Health status — general evaluation
      2) Symptoms of illness
      3) Disability days — bed days, restricted activity days, work-loss days, school-loss days (for at least two days in last 12 months), condition and duration of condition caused disability days and perceived seriousness of it
      4) Chronic activity limitation — condition that kept one from usual activity

       b. Evaluated

         1) Medically-defined need — diagnoses severity rating

         2) Diagnosis — conditions

         3) Surgery — operations

II.   OUTCOME INDICES

  A. *Utilization of Health Services*

    1. Type

      a. Hospital

      b. Physician — general practitioner, specialist, chiropractor

      c. Dentist

      d. Nursing and personal care homes

      e. Prescribed and nonprescribed drugs — druggist

      f. Home care

      g. Emergency care

      h. Other — x-rays, lab tests, visiting nurse or health aide, spiritualist or faith healer, nurse

    2. Site — home, office or private clinic; hospital inpatient, outpatient, emergency room; other clinic; telephone

    3. Purpose

      a. Preventive

         1) General exam — time interval and content

         2) Obstetrical — number and trimester of visits for pregnancy, family planning practices

      b. Illness-related

         1) Curative — acute disability

         2) Stabilizing — chronic disability

      c. Custodial

    4. Time interval

      a. Contact — did or did not see doctor (or other health worker) for condition in past 12 months; did or did not see dentist in past 12 months; was or was not admitted to hospital in past 12 months; etc.

      b. Volume — number of doctor, dentist visits; number of hospital admissions and length of stay; etc.

      c. Continuity — episodes of illness (by recency); first provider seen, number of visits for given episodes, same or different doctor for each visit; reason for seeing different doctor (if applicable); delay and reasons for delay

B. *Consumer Satisfaction*

Reasons cited for why people sometimes do not see a medical doctor when they should: didn't want to lose time or pay from work; worried that boss might think you were too sick to work; didn't think a doctor could help you; doctor or place didn't have office hours that were convenient

SELECTED REFERENCES:

Richardson, W. C.

1971 *Ambulatory Use of Physician's Services in Response to Illness Episodes in a Low-Income Neighborhood.* Research Series No. 29. Chicago: Center for Health Administration Studies, University of Chicago.

System Sciences, Inc.

1971 *Initial Analyses of Baseline Surveys for Neighborhood Health Centers.* Bethesda, Maryland: System Sciences, Inc.

PERSONS TO BE CONTACTED ABOUT DATA SOURCE:

Gerald Sparer
Health Services Evaluation Division
Bureau of Health Services Research and Evaluation
    (NCHSRD)
Parklawn Building
5600 Fishers Lane
Rockville, Maryland 20852

William C. Richardson, Ph.D., Director
Graduate Program in Health Services Administration and Planning
School of Public Health and Community Medicine
University of Washington
Seattle, Washington 97105

Division of Health Insurance Studies, Office of Research and Statistics, Social Security Administration (SSA), continuing reporting system on hospital and medical services covered by SSA

DESCRIPTION OF DATA SOURCE:

Times of collection (when and/or how often):

A continuing reporting system of statistics on utilization and charges for hospital and medical services covered by the Social

Security Administration and for the medical care providers of such services is maintained by the Division of Health Insurance Studies. The SSA's mandate for these continuing studies was part of the original (1935) Social Security Act.

In addition, to obtain information about the supplementary medical insurance programs under Medicare, monthly interviews of a five percent (5%) sample of the enrolled Medicare population are conducted in the Current Medicare Survey (CMS).

Population and/or sample:

All recipients and participating providers of hospital and medical services under the public assistance — and Medicare — based health insurance programs of the Social Security Administration provide the data for the ongoing data collection efforts.

Method of data collection:

Most of the information is obtained from patient and provider registration and claims records. The basic statistical system of the Medicare program, for example, is comprised of a health insurance entitlement master file, a central record of participating providers, hospital insurance (Part A) utilization record, medical insurance (Part B) payment record, and the record containing information from medical insurance bills for the five percent (5%) sample of supplementary medical insurance enrollees. The data on the five percent sample is obtained, however, from monthly personal interviews, using questionnaires and personal health care diaries.

RELEVANCE FOR THE STUDY OF ACCESS:

Though a variety of data are collected by the Office of Research and Statistics only the information relevant to the utilization and charges for covered services and provider characteristics will be summarized here. These data provide information, on a continuing basis, on the volume and kinds of utilization of the population enrolled in federally supported health insurance plans and the characteristics of the providers who render services to them. The system may well serve as a model for a national system of accounts on the utilization, expenditures and providers of services, participating in a program of universal national health insurance.

I.   PROCESS INDICES

    A. *Characteristics of Health Delivery System*

       1. Statistics relating to the characteristics of participating

providers of services to enrollees, such as hospitals, skilled nursing facilities, home health agencies, and independent laboratories, including analysis of terminations and changes over time.

2. Statistics measuring the progress of state agencies in certifying hospitals, skilled nursing facilities, home health agencies and independent clinical laboratories for participation in the health insurance program; statistics on the extent to which various types of health care facilities meet or fail to meet specific conditions of participating over time as well as on the number and characteristics of health care facilities whose certifications are terminated.

3. Variations within and between geographic areas in the distribution of facilities, range of services offered, availability of skilled technical personnel.

B. *Characteristics of Population-at-Risk*

   1. Predisposing
      a. Immutable
         1) Age
         2) Sex
         3) Race or ethnicity

   2. Enabling
      a. Mutable
         1) Insurance coverage — type of payer, extent of coverage, method of payment (including deductible and co-insurance provisions for Medicare)
         2) Price of services
      b. Immutable
         1) Region

   3. Need
      a. Evaluated
         1) Diagnosis
         2) Surgical procedures

II.   OUTCOME INDICES

A. *Utilization*

The following summaries of the health services utilization and cost data collected for public assistance and medicare recipients by the Office of Research and Statistics at SSA appear in that office's *Fiscal Year 1974-75 Work Plan:*

1. Public assistance programs
   a. Type and charges for covered medical care services used by the aged and the disabled under the hospital insurance program, including inpatient hospital care, outpatient services, care in skilled nursing facilities and home health services. For each category data include the number of admissions and discharges, admission and discharge rates, length of stay, number and rate of surgical procedures, diagnostic data, charges for services.
   b. Utilization of and charges for physicians' services, including the number and rate of services, place of service, nature of treatment, charges for services, and other covered medical services under the supplementary medical insurance program, including laboratory tests, prosthetic appliances and so forth.
   c. Trends in utilization and charges since the beginning of the program.
2. Medicare program
   a. Estimates of the number of medical services, place and type of service, charges for these medical services, potential reimbursement from SSA, and source of payment for the portion not covered by Medicare.
   b. Estimates of the use and costs of prescription drugs and other noncovered services such as payments for routine physical examinations, dental services, eyeglasses or eye examination, and hearing aids; and utilization of and estimated expenses incurred for the services of noncovered practitioners, such as optometrists, naturopaths, and Christian Science practitioners.

SELECTED REFERENCES:

Social Security Administration, Office of Research and Statistics
Health Insurance Statistics (current issues). Washington, D.C.: Social Security Administration, Office of Research and Statistics, U.S. Dept. HEW Publication No. (SSA) 74-11702.

1971 *Medicare: Health Insurance for the Aged, 1967, Section 1: Summary.* Washington: Social Security Administration, Office of Research and Statistics.

Monthly Benefit Statistics (current issues). Washington: Social Security Administration, Office of Research and Statistics, U.S. Dept. HEW Publication No. (SSA) 74-11703.

1973 *Office of Research and Statistics: Fiscal Year 1974-75 Work Plan.* Washington: Social Security Administration, Office of Research and Statistics.

PERSONS TO BE CONTACTED ABOUT DATA SOURCE:

John J. Carroll
Assistant Commissioner for Research and Statistics
Office of Research and Statistics
Social Security Administration
1875 Connecticut Avenue, N.W.
Washington, D.C. 20009

Dorothy P. Rice
Deputy Assistant Commissioner for Research and Statistics
Office of Research and Statistics
Social Security Administration
1875 Connecticut Avenue, N.W.
Washington, D.C. 20009

Howard West, Director
Division of Health Insurance Studies
Office of Research and Statistics
Social Security Administration
1875 Connecticut Avenue, N.W.
Washington, D.C. 20009

Division of Health Insurance Studies, Office of Research and Statistics, Social Security Administration (SSA), study of Medicaid enrollees

DESCRIPTION OF DATA SOURCE:

Times of collection (when and/or how often):
This study was conducted in 1974.

Population and/or sample:
Approximately nine (9) Health Maintenance Organizations (HMO's), in which AFDC and OAS Medicaid recipients are enrolled, were sampled. Samples from the HMO's were matched (by geographic area, age, and family size and composition) with a sample of non-HMO Medicaid recipients. Approximately 800

households (with an average of 1.2 persons per household) were interviewed.

Method of data collection:

Household interviews of family members will constitute the means of collecting information on the HMO and non-HMO enrollees.

RELEVANCE FOR THE STUDY OF ACCESS:

The purpose of this study is to compare the utilization, satisfaction and "accessibility" of HMO members and non-HMO Medicaid recipients. It solicits information on dimensions relevant to numerous aspects of our access framework. It may serve as an example of a way to evaluate the effect of different organizational forms on access.

I.   PROCESS INDICES

   A. *Characteristics of Health Delivery System*

     Some information was collected that describes the organizational differences between the HMO's sampled. Information on system differences was primarily solicited in the context of the "enabling" characteristics of the population-at-risk, however.

   B. *Characteristics of Population-at-Risk*

     1. Predisposing

       a. Mutable

         1) Knowledge and sources of health care information

         2) Stress and anxiety about health

       b. Immutable

         1) Age

         2) Sex

         3) Marital status

         4) Previous health behavior

         5) Education

         6) Race and ethnicity

         7) Family size and composition

         8) Residential mobility

     2. Enabling

       a. Mutable

         1) Socioeconomic status

2) Insurance coverage — type of payer, extent of coverage, method of payment
3) Price of medical services
4) Organization of services — HMO and non-HMO enrollees
5) Regular source of care
6) Ease of getting care — perceived time one must wait to see doctor for selected conditions, problems making appointment, waiting time for appointment, method of transportation to care, travel time to care, difficulty of travelling to care, arrangements for children to be taken care of while seeing doctor, office waiting time, waiting time for doctor to return telephone call

  b. Immutable
    1) Region
    2) Residence

3. Need
  a. Perceived
    1) Health status — general evaluation, worry
    2) Symptoms of illness — when symptoms first occurred
    3) Disability days — bed days in past three years and last year, restricted activity days in past three years and last year, condition and duration of condition causing disability days and bother associated with it
    4) Chronic activity limitation — condition that lasted more than three months
  b. Evaluated
    1) Diagnosis — conditions, accidents
    2) Surgery

II.   OUTCOME INDICES

  A. *Utilization*
    1. Type
      a. Hospital
      b. Physician
      c. Nursing and personal care homes
      d. Prescribed and nonprescribed drugs
      e. Appliances — vision and hearing aids

      f. Emergency care — emergency room, ambulance

      g. Other — x-rays, lab tests, para-medical personnel

2. Site — home; office or private clinic; hospital inpatient, outpatient, emergency room; neighborhood health center, school, or other clinic; telephone

3. Purpose

    a. Preventive

      1) General exam — time interval and reason

      2) Obstetrical — number and trimester of visits for pregnancy

    b. Illness-related

      1) Curative — acute conditions

      2) Stabilizing — chronic conditions

    c. Custodial

4. Time interval

    a. Contact — did or did not see doctor in past month; was or was not admitted to hospital in past year, etc.

    b. Volume — number of hospital admissions and length of stay; etc.

    c. Continuity — reason for patient going to particiular provider; delay and reasons for delay

B. *Consumer Satisfaction*

Level of satisfaction (for specific visit) with appointment waiting time, travel time, office waiting time, amount of time doctor spent with you, doctor's treatment of condition, doctor's explanation of problem, personal concern shown by doctor, completeness of exam, and, generally, with the care received; reasons cited for delaying to seek care from physician.

SELECTED REFERENCES:

Contact project director, listed below.

PERSON TO BE CONTACTED ABOUT DATA SOURCE:

Dr. Clifton R. Gaus
Division of Health Insurance Studies
Office of Research and Statistics
Social Security Administration
1875 Connecticut Avenue, N.W.
Washington, D.C. 20009

World Health Organization International Collaborative Study of Medical Care Utilization (WHO/ICS-MCU)

DESCRIPTION OF DATA SOURCE:

Times of collection (when and/or how often):

This survey was conducted throughout each of four quarters from June 1, 1968, to May 31, 1969. The study was conducted over a year's period of time, so that seasonal variations in disease, etc., in the different study areas would not compromise the comparability of the findings across areas.

Population and/or sample:

Samples were drawn in the following areas: Canada (Grande Prairie, Saskatchewan, Fraser and Jersey); United States (Northwestern Vermont, Baltimore); Argentina (Buenos Aires); United Kingdom (Liverpool); Finland (Helsinki); Poland (Lodz); and Yugoslavia (Banat, Rijeka). Because of the diversity of sampling information available to the different study areas, each area developed its sampling design to permit 1) calculation of population estimates, rates and standard errors of use with a specified degree of precision, and 2) within-area analyses of individuals by various statistical methods, including multivariate analysis. The number of persons interviewed ranged from 2,881 in Liverpool to 5,463 in Banat.

Methods of data collection:

Household interviews of the population-at-risk and descriptive assessments of the health services system and demography in an area comprised the data collection mechanisms.

RELEVANCE FOR THE STUDY OF ACCESS:

This study was conducted at a single point in time for a number of different delivery systems. The data from the different study areas permit comparisons of access across delivery systems.

I.   PROCESS INDICES

A. *Characteristics of Health Delivery System*

Information on the resources and organization of the delivery systems in the respective areas was systematically collected, separate from the data gathered through household interviews. The type of data collected in each area is summarized below:

1. Resources
   a. Ratios of physicians and number of hours available per 10,000 population
   b. Ratio of dentists, nurses, and other health workers per 10,000 population
   c. Short-stay and long-term hospital beds per 1,000 population
2. Organization
   a. System points of entry — number of points of entry at which services can be obtained without mandatory referral
   b. Financing — level of medical expenditures borne by the system
   c. Distributional responsibility — degree of formal responsibility for the optimal distribution of services
   d. Administrative requirements — general organization of the system administratively
   e. Drug dispensing policies — method of certifying eligibility for use of drugs
   f. Health indicators — indices of health status of population
   g. Public health indices — indicators of illegitimacy rate, venereal disease rate, etc.
   h. Economic indices — GNP, health economic indices, etc.

B. *Characteristics of Population-at-Risk*
   1. Predisposing
      a. Mutable
         1) General health care beliefs and attitudes — skepticism towards medicine, . . . toward doctors, dependency in illness, tendency to use services for somatic problems, . . . for psycho-social problems
         2) Knowledge and source of health care information
         3) Stress and anxiety about health
      b. Immutable
         1) Age
         2) Sex
         3) Marital status
         4) Previous health behavior — cigarette smoking
         5) Education
         6) Race or ethnicity

       7) Family size and composition — who is primarily responsible for health of family

  2. Enabling

    a. Mutable

      1) Socioeconomic status and occupation

      2) Income and sources of income

      3) Insurance coverage — varied by study area

      4) Price of medical services

      5) Organization of services — collected on system-level

      6) Regular source of care

      7) Ease of getting to care — method of transportation, travel time, appointment or walk-in visit, appointment waiting time, office waiting time

      8) Availability of health resources — collected on system-level

    b. Immutable

      1) Region — study area

      2) Residence

  3. Need

    a. Perceived

      1) Health status — general evaluation, worry, pain, severity index, dental, morbidity index

      2) Symptoms of illness — phlegm, pain in joints, shortness of breath

      3) Disability days — bed days, restricted activity days in two weeks, condition and duration of condition causing disability days and perceived seriousness of it

      4) Chronic activity limitation — physical impairment, visual defect

    b. Evaluated

      1) Medically-defined need — angina pectoris, rheumatoid arthritis, breathlessness, chronic bronchitis

      2) Diagnosis — conditions

II.   OUTCOME INDICES

  A. *Utilization of Health Services*

    1. Type

    a. Hospital

        b. Physician — medical doctor, chiropractor, foot doctor, optometrist (or optician)

        c. Dentist

        d. Nursing and personal care homes

        e. Prescribed and nonprescribed drugs — druggist

        f. Appliances — vision aids

        g. Emergency care

        h. Other — healer, midwife, nurse

2. Site — other; office or private clinics; hospital inpatient, outpatient, emergency room; industrial or school clinic; well-baby clinic; other clinic; telephone

3. Purpose

        a. Preventive

           1) General and vision exams — time interval, reason, location

           2) Immunizations — time interval, location

        b. Illness-related

           1) Curative — acute illness

           2) Stabilizing — chronic illness

        c. Custodial

4. Time interval

        a. Contact — did or did not see a doctor (or other health workers) in two weeks (for condition); did or did not see dentist in past month; was or was not admitted to hospital in past year; etc.

        b. Volume — number of doctor, dentist visits; number of hospital admissions and length of stay; etc.

        c. Continuity — person who suggested most recent contact with medical care provider, if anyone; delay and reason for delay

B. *Consumer Satisfaction*

Level of satisfaction (for most recent M.D. contact) with appointment waiting time, office waiting time, time physician spent with you, and what happened at that consultation; level of satisfaction (for usual source of care) with convenience of location and office hours; perceived availability of care (in general) based on whether or not the respondent thought it was easy to get to see a doctor at night, was too much trouble to see a doctor, one had to wait too long to see a doctor, and whether it was easy to see a doctor during his office hours;

reasons cited (when disability days were reported in past two weeks) for not consulting a doctor — did not want to, did not have time to go, too much trouble, etc.

SELECTED REFERENCES:

Rabin, D. L. (ed.)

> 1972 "International comparisons of medical care." *Milb. Mem. Fund Quart* 50 (July): 1-99.

WHO/ICS-MCU

> 1970 *WHO/ICS-MCU Manuals 1-9.* Baltimore: WHO/ICS-MCU Coordinating Committee, Department of Medical Care and Hospitals, Johns Hopkins University.
> 1. Organization and development
> 2. Questionnaires
> 3. Health services systems and demography
> 4. Training and supervisors' manual
> 5. Interviewers' manual
> 6. Coders' manual
> 7. Analysis manual
> 8. Tape layout manual
> 9. Data processing manual

PERSONS TO BE CONTACTED ABOUT DATA SOURCE:

Project Directors

Donald O. Anderson, M.D., S.M. in Hyg., F.R.C.P. (C) Professor
Department of Health Care and Epidemiology
University of British Columbia
Room 300, Wesbrook Building
Vancouver 8, British Columbia
Canada

Ivo Brodarec, M.D., Director
Institute of Public Health of Croatia
Rockefellerova 7, Zagreb
Yugoslavia

Stanley Greenhill, M.D.
Professor and Chairman
Department of Community Medicine
13-108 Clinical Science Building
University of Alberta
Edmonton 7, Alberta
Canada

Janusz Indulski, M.D., Director
Department of Health Care Organization
Akademia Medyczna W Lodz
ul. Narutowicza Nv. 96
Lodz
Poland

Robert F. L. Logan, M.D., F.R.C.P.
Professor of Organization of Medical Care
London School of Hygiene and Tropical Medicine
University of London
Keppel Street, Gower Street
London, W.C.1
England

John H. Mabry, Ph.D., Professor
Department of Community Medicine
Given Building
University of Vermont
Burlington, Vermont 05401

Vincent L. Matthews, M.D., D.P.H.
Professor and Head
Department of Social and Preventive Medicine
236 Medical Building
Saskatoon, Saskatchewan
Canada

Jose Maria Paganini, M.D., M.P.H.
Project Director, WHO/ICS-MCU
Encuesta de Salud
Hospital Escuela "Jose de San Martin"
Cordoba 2351 - Piso 11
Buenos Aires, Argentina
South America

Tapani Purola, Dr. Pol. Sc., Director
Research Institute for Social Security
National Pensions Institute
Nordenskioldinkatu 12
Helsinki 25
Finland

David L. Rabin, M.D., M.P.H.
Associate Professor
Department of Medical Care and Hospitals
School of Hygiene and Public Health
The Johns Hopkins University
615 North Wolfe Street
Baltimore, Maryland 21205

Cedomir Vukmanovic, M.D.
Assistant Director
Federal Institute of Public Health
Slobodana Penezica 35
Belgrade
Yugoslavia

health
administration
press

M2240 School of Public Health
The University of Michigan
Ann Arbor, Michigan 48104
(313) 764-1380

Lewis E. Weeks, Ph.D.
Editor

The Press was founded in 1972 with the support of the W. K. Kellogg Foundation as a joint endeavor of the Association of University Programs in Health Administration and the Cooperative Information Center for Hospital Management Studies.

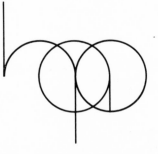